ABBREVIATIONS

M	—mass
min	—minute
mm	—millimeter
mmHg	—millimeters of mercury
MPA	—main pulmonary artery
m/s	—meters per second
MV	—mitral valve
P	—posterior
	—pulmonary valve
	—pericardium
	—pulmonary artery
PA	—pulmonary artery
PDA	—patent ductus arteriosus
PE	—pleural effusion
	—pericardial effusion
PGE$_1$	—prostaglandin E$_1$
PI	—pulmonary insufficiency
PL	—posterior ledge
PS	—pulmonary stenosis
PT	—pulmonary trunk
PV	—pulmonary valve
PVal	—pulmonary valve
PVC	—pulmonary venous confluence
R	—right
RA	—right atrium
RAA	—right atrial appendage
RB-T	—right Blalock-Taussig shunt
RCA	—right carotid artery
RIA	—right innominate artery
R-L	—right to left
RL	—right lung
RLL	—right lower lobe
RML	—right middle lobe

RMLA	—right-sided morphologic left atrium
RPA	—right pulmonary artery
RPDA	—right patent ductus arteriosus
RSA	—right subclavian artery
RSVC	—right superior vena cava
Rt Arch	—right-sided aortic arch
RUL	—right upper lobe
RUPV	—right upper pulmonary vein
RV	—right ventricle
RVOC	—right ventricular subaortic outlet chamber
RVOT	—right ventricular outflow tract
s	—second
S	—spine
	—superior
	—systolic component
	—systole
SA	—subclavian artery
SMA	—superior mesenteric artery
SVC	—superior vena cava
t	—trachea
T	—tunnel
	—overriding truncus
	—thrombosis
	—teratoma
TD	—thermal dilution
TH	—tubular hypoplasia
TV	—tricuspid valve
TVI	—time velocity integral
V	—ventricle
VA	—vertebral artery
VS	—ventricular septum
VSD	—ventricular septal defect

PEDIATRIC IMAGING/
DOPPLER ULTRASOUND
OF THE CHEST:
EXTRACARDIAC DIAGNOSIS

PEDIATRIC IMAGING/ DOPPLER ULTRASOUND OF THE CHEST: EXTRACARDIAC DIAGNOSIS

James C. Huhta, M.D.

Associate Professor of Pediatrics
Baylor College of Medicine
Associate in Pediatric Cardiology and
Director of Echocardiography Laboratory
Texas Children's Hospital
Houston, Texas

Illustrations by Timothy H. Phelps, M.S.

Lea & Febiger

Philadelphia

1986

Lea & Febiger
600 Washington Square
Philadelphia, PA   19106-4198
U.S.A.
(215) 922-1330

Supported in part by: Grant G-410 from the American Heart Association, Texas Affiliate;
New Investigator Research Award HL31153 from the National Heart, Lung, and Blood
Institute, National Institutes of Health, United States Public Health Service; Grant RR-
05425 from the National Institutes of Health, United States Public Health Service; and
Grant RR-00188 from the General Clinical Research Branch, National Institutes of Health,
United States Public Health Service.

Library of Congress Cataloging-in-Publication Data

Huhta, James.
  Pediatric imaging/Doppler ultrasound of the chest.

  Includes bibliographies and index.
  1. Ultrasonic cardiography. 2. Pediatric cardiology—
Diagnosis. 3. Chest—Diseases—Diagnosis. I. Title.
[DNLM: 1. Thoracic Diseases—diagnosis. 2. Thoracic
Diseases—in infancy & childhood. 3. Ultrasonic
Diagnosis—in infancy & childhood. WF 975 H989p]
RJ423.5.U46H84   1986   618.92'0975407543   86-2806
ISBN 0-8121-1037-4

PRINTED IN THE UNITED STATES OF AMERICA

Print number: 5 4 3 2 1

*To the Glory of God,
and to Nancy, My Wife*

FOREWORD

In 1977, author-echocardiographers Howard Gutgesell and Marc Paquet asked me to write a foreword for their book on the M-mode echocardiogram in congenital heart malformations, *Atlas of Pediatric Echocardiography.* I did so reluctantly, since I had never touched a transducer, and probably, as a result, never really understood the M-mode echocardiogram. (I had been told by these two self-taught experts, while they were in my training program, that it was dangerous for a man of my age to stand too close to the new echo equipment!) What pediatric echo pioneers Gutgesell and Paquet put together became a widely used handbook that guided many a budding echocardiographer in deciphering the single dimensional ultrasonic mysteries that emanated from a myriad of congenital cardiac defects.

During the past few years, advanced ultrasound technology has relegated the M-mode recording equipment to the diagnosis of pericardial effusion and measurement of shortening fractions and systolic time intervals. (In the meantime, however, Gutgesell and Paquet seem to have escaped such confined relegation themselves, and each has moved on to the lofty heights of division chief in a pediatric cardiology center.) Inevitably, two-dimensional views, like two heads, proved to be better than one; furthermore, Doppler technique made the analysis of transvalvular blood flow, velocity, and direction possible, and gave clinicians the information in numbers that they had been hearing for decades with their stethoscopes. It also became evident, through this advanced technology, that there are some Doppler-detectable events in the cardiac cycle that the clinician cannot hear at all. These new methods stimulated the interest of the nonultrasonic clinician who had been baffled long enough by the unfamiliar M-mode images. The nonultrasonic clinician now began to see in the two-dimensional picture something that looked like the familiar angiocardiogram, or a selected slice through a dissected specimen in the pathology laboratory.

The appointment of James Huhta to our faculty in 1982 coincided with our purchase of two-dimensional ultrasound and Doppler equipment. Armed with one degree in electrical engineering, another in bioengineering, a fellowship in pediatric cardiology and, finally, a research year in pathologic-angiographic-echocardiographic comparisons, Huhta immediately set to work studying virtually every known heart anomaly in our patients who had heart catheterization.

He soon learned, to his satisfaction and evidently to that of peer review journals, when the technology, as well as the echocardiographer, could be relied upon to provide the surgeon with a definitive and noninvasive preoperative diagnosis.

There is no more staunch advocate of children than James Huhta, and he has found the ideal means to express this by so resolutely promoting the noninvasive diagnostic methods. The reader of this book will learn both the limitations and the values of these techniques in the diagnosis of intrathoracic diseases and anomalies.

Houston, Texas   Dan G. McNamara, M.D.

PREFACE

This book is intended for use by all those caring for children with diseases of the chest—cardiologists, pediatricians, radiologists, and surgeons. The student of diagnostic ultrasound will find a summary of chest disorders present in patients ranging in age from 1 day to 20 years, and in weight from 500 g to 80 kg. From a large clinical experience at Texas Children's Hospital, this book presents a practical, step-by-step method of noninvasive diagnosis of: (1) extracardiac anatomy with high resolution ultrasound imaging and (2) vascular blood flow assessment with Doppler techniques.

It is my intention that this text be one from which the student already familiar with gross thoracic anatomy may acquaint himself with a tomographic, segmental approach to diagnosis of extracardiac abnormalities. If he possesses some knowledge of cardiovascular hemodynamics, the reader will gain an introduction to noninvasive blood flow velocity measurement using Doppler techniques.

Standard views of the aorta and the pulmonary and systemic veins are presented with illustrations of a wide range of abnormalities—congenital and acquired. New information is presented regarding the application of ultrasound to day-to-day clinical problems in pediatrics, such as assessment of the diaphragm function, diagnosis of pleural effusion, masses in the chest, and the use of imaging/Doppler ultrasound in the intensive care unit for the measurement of cardiac function in neonates and children.

For the cross-sectional ultrasonic images a consistent method of figure labeling is used, giving a rough orientation to the tomographic plane and the nearby important structures. Common projection planes and a comparison with other radiographic techniques are reviewed in Chapter 2. Doppler illustrations showing a blood flow velocity waveform are labeled with an orientation to the direction of sampling, usually with a corresponding image. The figure abbreviations are summarized on the front endpapers.

I hope that this book will increase the use of the tools and techniques of ultrasound in the management of pediatric disorders of the chest.

Houston, Texas   James C. Huhta, M.D.

ACKNOWLEDGMENTS

This book would not have been possible without the encouragement and support of Dan G. McNamara, M.D. Many others contributed to the patient data collection that supported this effort, including Dr. Howard P. Gutgesell, Dr. Daniel J. Murphy, Dr. David Danford, our pediatric cardiology fellows, and the Texas Children's Hospital Echocardiography Laboratory staff, particularly F. Douglas Huffines, RDMS, Heidi Elder, Lucy Tabrizi, Regina Hanson, Susan Russo, and Michelle Shotlow.

I am indebted to Timothy Phelps for the artwork, to Dr. Deborah Kearney, of the Department of Pathology, Baylor College of Medicine, for the pathology examples, and to Dr. Robert Morrow, Fellow in Pediatric Cardiology, for permission to present the quantitative data on the aortic arch.

Manuscript review and many helpful comments were contributed by Dr. Wesly Vick III, Drs. Ali Khan and Saad Al-Youset at the Military Hospital, Riyadh, Saudi Arabia, Dr. Robert Dutton in the Department of Radiology at Texas Children's Hospital, and Drs. Daniel J. Murphy and Arthur T. Garson of the Lillie Frank Abercrombie Section of Pediatric Cardiology, Department of Pediatrics, Baylor College of Medicine.

I would like to extend my appreciation to Lea & Febiger, in particular to Kenneth Bussy and Thomas Colaiezzi for their assistance. Nancy Mitchell typed the references, figure legends, and Chapter 8, and the Apple Macintosh computer did the rest.

J.C.H.

CONTENTS

chapter 1

TECHNIQUES OF THE PEDIATRIC ULTRASOUND EXAMINATION

Noninvasive techniques have great appeal to pediatricians, whose unwritten charge in clinical medicine includes advocacy for the patient who cannot speak for himself. Ultrasound imaging and Doppler assessment have had a major impact on the discipline of pediatrics, particularly pediatric cardiology. Some believe that noninvasive imaging has been the most significant advance in the last decade in the care of patients with congenital heart disease; it ranks with the therapeutic use of prostaglandins and interventional catheterization laboratory techniques. In the days before ultrasound, the possibility of ductus-dependent circulation in the critically ill neonate could be settled only by cardiac catheterization and angiography. The once difficult distinction between total anomalous pulmonary venous connection and hyaline membrane disease (in the past resolved all too often by the pathologist) is now a relatively straightforward task for the echocardiographer, who can identify the normal or abnormal connection of the pulmonary veins.

The use of ultrasonography for the diagnosis of extracardiac abnormalities of the chest in children has received little attention. When performed in an organized and step-by-step fashion, ultrasound of the chest complements standard radiographic techniques and sometimes provides a definitive diagnosis. The extent to which ultrasound benefits patient care depends primarily on the skill of the examiner who performs each study. We hope to expand the application of diagnostic ultrasound in the child with known or possible extracardiac problems within the chest.

THE SEGMENTAL APPROACH

Originally described by Van Praagh,[1] the segmental approach to congenital heart disease forms the basis of cardiac anatomic diagnosis. At the Texas Children's Hospital Echocardiography Laboratory, we have expanded this approach to include extracardiac anatomy of the chest. The chapter titles of this book outline a summary of this concept, which is necessary when applying any tomographic method of imaging to the thorax.

For the purposes of this approach, the aorta consists of four segments: ascending, arch, isthmus, and descending. Pulmonary arteries and veins are individually examined. Systemic venous segments are sequentially imaged. Noncardiovascular structures such as the diaphragm, the thymus, and the esophagus are each examined in turn. Even with the expected advent of three-dimensional imaging in ultrasonography, a logical sequence in chest imaging will be vital to a high quality result. The future will bring many changes in technology, but the foundation of diagnosis will remain knowing the anatomy, what abnormalities may occur, and how they appear tomographically.

PEDIATRIC EXAMINATION

Our goal is to present a systematic, segmental method for the evaluation of the extracardiac anatomy. No noninvasive test such as ultrasound can replace

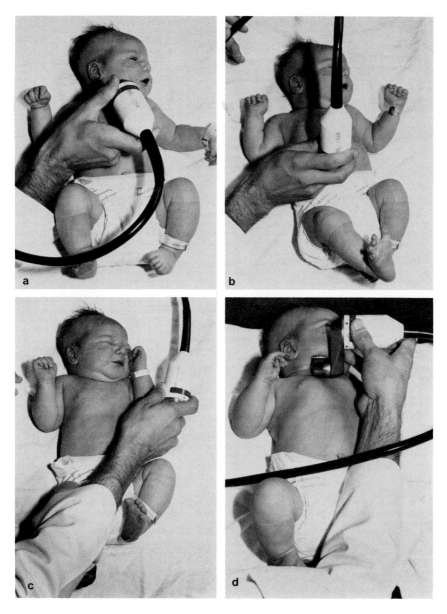

FIG. 1–1. Ultrasonic windows that can be utilized in the newborn and the infant for examination of extracardiac structures. (a) Supine position with parasternal scanning, (b) subcostal scanning in a coronal plane, (c) apical four-chamber position, and (d) suprasternal scanning.

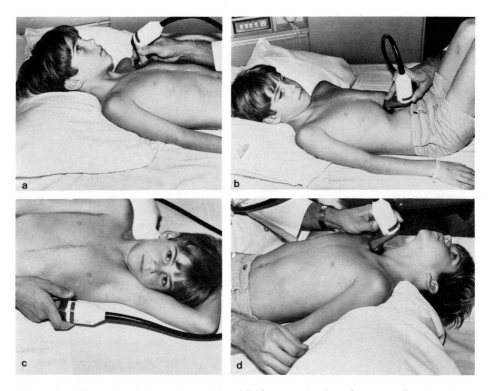

FIG. 1–2.   Ultrasonic windows in an older child for examination of extracardiac structures. (a) Parasternal scans, (b) subcostal scans, (c) apical scans, and (d) suprasternal scans.

the observations of the experienced clinician. The ideal marriage is the use of ultrasonography by the clinician to solve patient problems. Ultrasound equipment soon will become a routine part of the clinical examination of a child with disease of the chest. The clinical experience described in this book spans a period of three years and includes over 10,000 examinations; it is intended to portray ultrasonography as a clinical tool.

Ultrasonic examination of the chest is limited by the interposition of inflated lung between the chest wall and the structure being examined, but it is possible in the pediatric age group because of fairly constant ultrasound "windows." These provide access for ultrasound waves to penetrate the interior of the chest and to scan the extracardiac structures. These four windows are the parasternal, the subcostal, the apical, and the suprasternal approaches. Depending upon the degree of inflation of the lungs, most of the extracardiac structures of the chest can be imaged by ultrasound by combining information from all of these approaches (Figure 1–1). However, the diagnostic approach should be based on a structure-oriented technique with scans from one area to another. In order to image all the structures of the chest, it is imperative to avoid the temptation to be "view-oriented" in the pediatric examination. An abnormality on one view must be confirmed on several scans from different positions. The feasibility of such an examination in children was demonstrated by our results in imaging the aorta in a consecutive series of children.[2] All the aortic segments could be evaluated in 98% of infants and children and each segment could be studied.

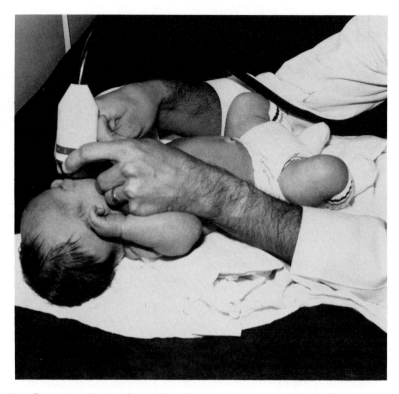

FIG. 1–3. Scanning of an infant using the suprasternal approach. Note that the suprasternal notch is exposed by placing a roll behind the shoulders of the infant so that the head falls back gently and the transducer is steadied in the suprasternal notch. Both of the operator's elbows are placed on the table to avoid discomfort to the infant from unintentional pressure to the neck.

This is in contrast to the poor feasibility of this type of extracardiac diagnosis in adults[3] and emphasizes the relative underutilization of ultrasonography in pediatric thoracic problems.

The sequence of steps in the examination of the older child is similar to that in the adult (Figure 1–2). The following is a summary of the methods that are used for diagnosis during a routine examination of extracardiac anatomy in our laboratory at Texas Children's Hospital.

1. Parasternal—transverse and sagittal scans along the sternum and under the clavicles, including examination of the great arteries and veins.
2. Subcostal—transverse and coronal scans from the abdomen, including determination of atrial situs, side of the cardiac apex, and visualization of the diaphragm and posterior mediastinum.
3. Apical—sagittal and coronal scans from the cardiac apex, including localization of the origin of the aorta and the pulmonary arteries.
4. Suprasternal—coronal and sagittal scans from above the sternum and clavicles for visualization and Doppler sampling of the aorta, superior venous return, and anterior mediastinum.

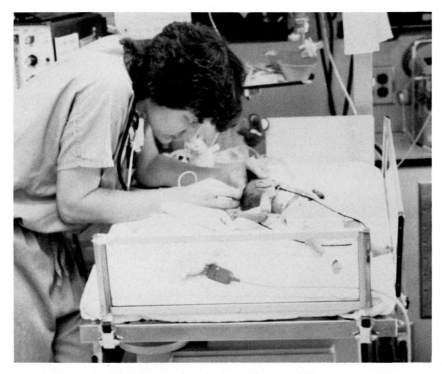

FIG. 1–4. Example of the examination situation for a premature infant. An open warmer allows access to the child for various procedures and for ultrasonic examination.

ULTRASOUND EQUIPMENT

Ultrasound equipment for use with pediatric patients has requirements that are substantially different from those for noninvasive imaging in adults. Because the infant and child tend to be more active during the examination, the equipment must be designed to allow ready access to front panel knobs and switching controls. Often two hands are required to steady the transducer on a baby so that no pressure is applied to the infant during the test. The examiner's elbows are placed on the table (Figure 1–3). Liberal use of foot pedals is helpful for the examiner, such as for switching to the Doppler mode. Doppler examination can be performed simultaneously with cross-sectional imaging using newer ultrasound equipment. Even with such capability, it may be difficult to obtain high quality Doppler records in a squirming child. Some authors prefer to use the Doppler methods without imaging, and with experience and a prior knowledge of the anatomy from a previous complete cross-sectional examination, this can be accomplished (see Chapter 3).

Examination of the critically ill child or newborn must be carried out in the intensive care setting. This places special requirements on the equipment configuration regarding portability, power requirements and connectors, and the usual engineering design considerations concerning leakage of current and shock hazard. The use of an "open warmer" allows access to the small infant for the examination (Figure 1–4). It is important for the examiner to be aware of the

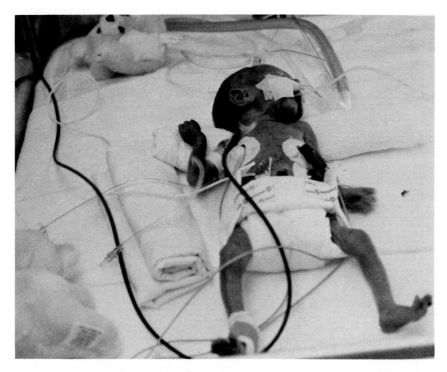

FIG. 1–5. The examiner must be aware of the various support systems for the critically ill infant, including the endotracheal tube, intravenous lines, temperature measuring devices, and the electrocardiograph. Some of these must be temporarily disconnected or rearranged in order to perform the complete ultrasonic examination.

child's support systems, such as the endotracheal tube and ventilator attachments, so that the examination can be carried out without causing harm to the child (Figure 1–5).

TRANSDUCERS

Because smaller structures are being examined, it is necessary to use ultrasound transducers of very high frequency such as 5, 7, or 10 mHz. It is possible to image with such frequencies because the depth of imaging is less, and the limitation of increasing attenuation of ultrasound energy at higher frequencies is balanced by the smaller size and depth of the subject. Imaging in premature infants may require frequencies up to 10 mHz, but in older children and adolescents a lower frequency transducer such as is used for adult examinations usually is entirely adequate.

The *shape* of the transducer is of importance in pediatric ultrasound work, especially when the subcostal and suprasternal notch approaches are used. The transducer head should not have any sharp or irregular edges that might cause discomfort and make the examination more difficult. In order to avoid excessive pressure on the abdomen or neck, it is helpful to have a transducer head designed to image at right angles to the plane of the transducer body (Figure 1–6). The

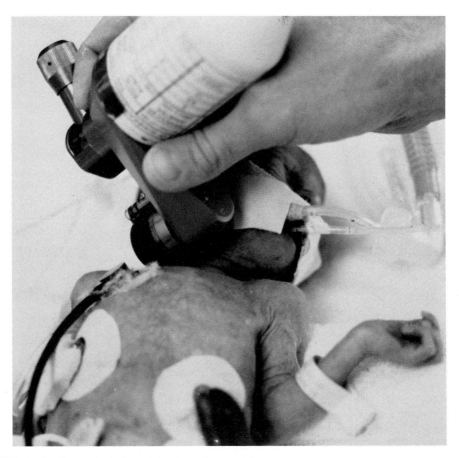

FIG. 1–6. Suprasternal examination of a critcally ill premature infant using a transducer from Advanced Technology Laboratories with an offset configuration that allows a steep angle of imaging from the suprasternal notch appproach.

size of the transducer is also important because it must fit into the neck and subxiphoid areas of even small infants.

PATIENT POSITIONING

Most ultrasound scans of the chest are performed with the patient in the supine position (Figure 1–7). The left lateral position will often enhance the quality of parasternal scans. Subcostal or Doppler imaging is aided by having the patient raise his or her knees. A pillow or folded towel behind the patient's shoulders will aid in gaining access to the suprasternal notch. It is important to avoid pressure on the child's neck by supporting the transducer with two hands and by placing one's elbows on the examining table or supporting one's hands on the patient's chest.

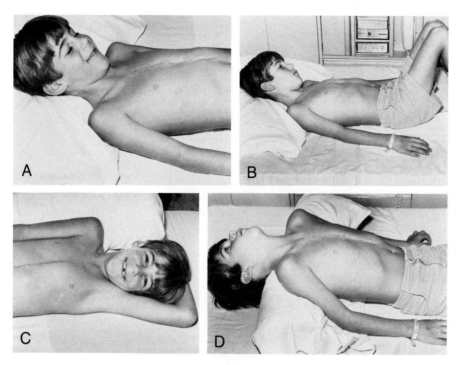

FIG. 1–7. A–D: Examples of various patient positions for ultrasound scanning.

ULTRASOUND WINDOWS FOR EXTRACARDIAC IMAGING

There is little information available concerning the usable portions of the chest for ultrasonography in the infant and child. Though ultrasound access is limited in pediatric patients with illnesses that cause lung overinflation, such as obstructive airway disease, or in those on assisted ventilation, the ultrasound windows are relatively large. In a preliminary attempt to obtain this information in normals, we measured the regions of ultrasonic access to the thorax in infants and children of different ages (Figure 1–8), and nearly the entire left chest could be used.

PARASTERNAL

Because of continuity of the heart and the pleuropericardial unit anteriorly, there is access to the mediastinum along the sternum (Figure 1–2a). The parasternal ultrasound window extends into the neck and to the left of the sternum. Because of intermittent intervening lung at the lower sternal border, changes in patient position should be routine during the ultrasonic examination. Parasternal scanning will be improved in most children and even in infants by utilizing the left lateral decubitus position. Slight rotation of the child to the left or right allows a more extensive examination.

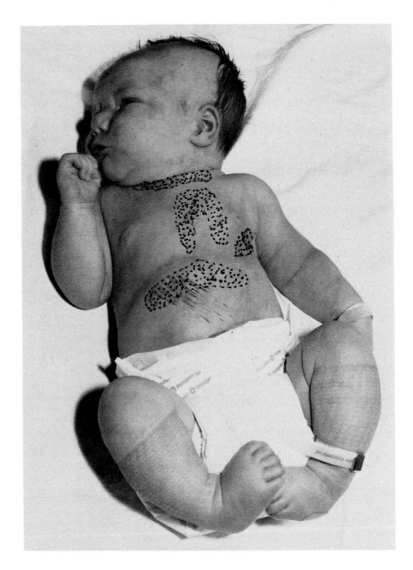

FIG. 1–8. Windows for ultrasonic energy transmission over the chest in an infant. Note the extension of the parasternal window over the region of the cardiac apex with a quiet, supine infant.

SUBCOSTAL

Subcostal (or subxiphoid) ultrasonic access is more than one transducer position immediately below the xiphoid process (Figure 1–2b). When performing coronal scanning it is important to position the transducer low in the abdomen. Imaging here is limited only by the possible interference of air-filled bowel. Scanning from below the right and left costal margins is important to detect pleural effusion but also to evaluate the diaphragm (see Chapter 12). Deep inspiration that is held will bring the diaphragm down and improve visualization of more superior structures from this approach in a cooperative older child.

Subcostal sagittal scanning of the mediastinum is performed aiming superiorly, with the transducer rotated 90 degrees to the subcostal coronal plane. Complete subcostal examination has been explained in detail by workers from Boston Children's Hospital.[4]

APICAL

With the patient in the left lateral decubitus position, the cardiac mass is displaced toward the chest wall, allowing ultrasonic examination from this region (Figure 1–2c). Scanning from a posterior to an anterior direction, the atria, ventricles, and great arteries are successively imaged. The pericardium and lateral cardiac walls are well visualized from this approach. Complete or partial exhalation will improve the apical window by reducing the amount of lung expansion around the cardiac apex.

SUPRASTERNAL

The extent of accessibility of the "suprasternal notch" approach is highly dependent on patient positioning and patient cooperation.[5,6] If possible, it is useful to have the patient exhale during parts of this test. Forced neck extension will only result in patient discomfort, and it is preferable to provide a pillow or rolled towel under the shoulders. The natural neck extension that results from the head's falling back over the pillow allows the suprasternal window to be utilized, and movement of the transducer to either side of the neck may result in good visualization of the superior mediastinum (Figure 1–2d).

THE NEONATE AND INFANT: SPECIAL CONSIDERATIONS

The ultrasonic examination of the neonate and infant must be tailored to the size, location, and clinical condition of the patient. Imaging quality in the neonate is superior because of the ultrasound windows. However, in the examination of a newborn infant, in order to avoid compromising the child, attention must be paid to the temperature of the environment, length of the examination, and

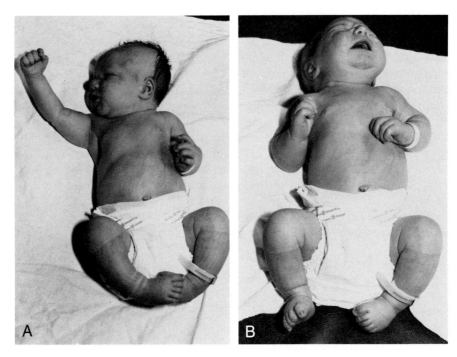

FIG. 1–9.   A and B: Examples of positioning of an infant for ultrasonic examination. Proper positioning will often hasten the achievement of good ultrasonic images and significantly shorten the examination. A roll behind the infant's shoulders will assist in obtaining scans from the suprasternal notch (B).

the examination technique. Attention to the positioning of the infant for the test will speed the examination (Figure 1–9). This is most important when examining a premature infant. In this situation, the simple application of pressure to the chest may cause bradycardia or respiratory difficulty.

A detail of the examination at the bedside of a seriously ill infant that cannot be overemphasized is providing a place for the examiner to sit down. This allows a minimum of disturbance to the infant and increases the possibility of a complete examination by decreasing operator fatigue.

In older infants between 6 and 30 months of age, the activity of the child will limit what can be done without sedation, and the goals of the test must be clearly defined before the examination is begun. It is useful to have an assistant entertain the child with a toy or doll in order to gain uninterrupted time. Bottle feeding should be done with care when the infant is in the recumbent position but is useful during suprasternal examination of the chest for visualization of the esophagus (see Chapter 4).

An anxious infant or toddler should be sedated when there are no contraindications such as severe respiratory distress in order to obtain a complete examination. We prefer oral administration of chloral hydrate in doses of 50 to 70 mg/kg body weight approximately one-half hour prior to the test. Frequently it is helpful to leave a frightened infant in the mother's lap during most of the examination (Figure 1–10).

The subcostal and suprasternal portions of the examination cause the most

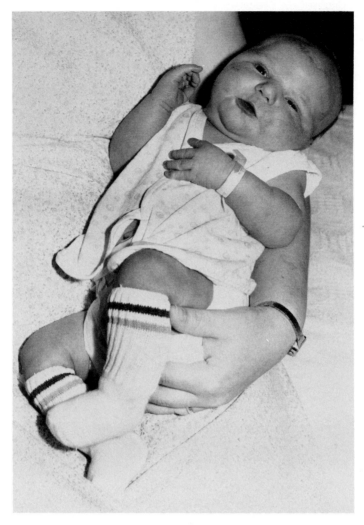

FIG. 1–10. Anxious infants may be optimally examined while in their mother's lap, where they are most comfortable.

irritation to an infant, and therefore we attempt to obtain as much information as possible from other ultrasound windows early in the examination. In such a child the typical order of examination outlined earlier would be modified to complete the most important parts of the test first. Beginning with the parasternal examination, the extracardiac aspects of the aorta, main pulmonary artery, and the systemic and pulmonary venous return can be imaged. The usual Doppler examination can be modified to utilize the parasternal and apical windows early in the examination.

REFERENCES

1. Van Praagh R: The segmental approach to diagnosis in congenital heart disease. *In* Bergsma D (ed): Birth Defects. Original Article Series Vol. 8, No. 5. Baltimore, Williams & Wikins, 1972, p. 4.

2. Huhta JC, Gutgesell HP, Latson LA, and Huffines FD: Two-dimensional echocardiographic assessment of the aorta in infants and children with congenital heart disease. Circulation, 70:417, 1984.
3. Bansal AC, Tajik AI, Seward JB, and Offord KP: Feasibility of detailed two-dimensional echocardiographic examination in adults. Prospective study of 200 patients. Mayo Clin Proc 55:291, 1980.
4. Sanders SP, Bierman FZ, and Williams RG: Conotruncal malformations: Diagnosis in infancy using subxiphoid 2-dimensional echocardiography. Am J Cardiol 50:1361, 1982.
5. Allen HD, Goldberg SJ, Sahn, DJ, et al: Suprasternal notch echocardiography: Assessment of its clinical utility in pediatric cardiology. Circulation 55:605, 1977.
6. Snider AR, and Silverman NH: Suprasternal notch echocardiography: A two-dimensional technique for evaluating congenital heart disease. Circulation 63:165, 1981.

chapter 2

CROSS-SECTIONAL ULTRASOUND IMAGING OF THE CHEST: A TOMOGRAPHIC APPROACH TO EXTRACARDIAC DIAGNOSIS

A tomographic approach to the structures of the chest using cross-sectional ultrasound imaging must be "structure-oriented" rather than view- or projection-oriented. The largest experience in pediatric ultrasound imaging of the chest has been directed toward the definition of intracardiac anatomy. Because of its unusual and lateralized position in the chest, the heart requires a unique set of tomographic views. Their orientation, dictated in part by the ultrasonic windows of the chest (see further on), is aligned with the long and short axis planes of the heart (Plate I). These standardized projections (including the long axis view, the short axis view, and the four-chamber view) effectively scan the intracardiac structures of importance, including the atria, ventricles, atrioventricular valves, semilunar valves, and intracardiac septa. Echocardiographic diagnosis of normal and abnormal intracardiac anatomy has been well described.[1-3] The purpose of this discussion is to illustrate the use of cross-sectional ultrasonography in the diagnosis of abnormalities of <u>extracardiac</u> anatomy in the chest.

TRANSVERSE SCANS

Structures in the chest that are outside the heart are best imaged using standard projection planes. *Transverse* images of the chest are utilized for routine chest radiography, computed axial tomography (CAT) scans, and nuclear magnetic resonance imaging. These planes, oriented perpendicular to the spine, are cross-sectional scans of the chest and are displayed as if one were sitting at the patient's feet and looking toward the head (Plate II). The patient's left is to the right and the anterior chest wall is superior. While ultrasonic images can be obtained in the midline over much of the chest, cephalad-caudad registration of these images is more difficult with ultrasound than with other methods because of the "sector" nature of most ultrasound imaging systems and the limited number of locations over the sternum where high-quality images can be obtained.

Transverse sections at the level of T8–10, just below the diaphragm, are useful for imaging the aorta and inferior vena cava in cross-section. The position of these two structures with respect to the spine is useful in the diagnosis of abnormalities of the atrial situs (Figure 2–1).[4,5] In asplenia syndrome, the inferior vena cava and aorta run together at this level. This scan is useful early in the examination to direct the examiner to exclude intra- and extracardiac abnormalities associated with abnormal atrial situs such as common atrium. With this scan, azygos vein continuation of the inferior vena cava can be diagnosed (see Chapter 11). Transverse scans below the sternum (subcostal) can be used to image the diaphragm and assess its function (see Chapter 12).

Higher on the sternum a transverse scan may be used to examine the position of the ascending aorta, the descending aorta, and the trachea. A transverse scan at the level of the aortic valve produces an oblique projection of the valve and the aorta and is not particularly useful for diagnosis of abnormalities. The atrial appendages may be visualized in such a scan and may be useful in the definition of atrial situs (see Chapter 11). High transverse scans will image the transverse aortic arch and the brachiocephalic arteries and veins. Although such scans closely resemble the CAT scan appearance of thoracic anatomy, as in all ultrasound imaging it is always preferable to be structure-oriented rather than view-oriented, even if it means deviating from standard planes.

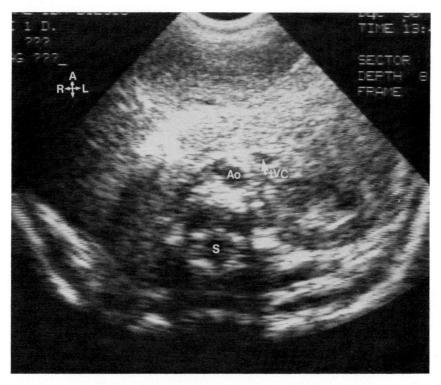

FIG. 2–1. Transverse ultrasonic scan of the abdomen showing the position of the spine (S), the aorta (Ao), and the inferior vena cava (IVC) in a patient with asplenia syndrome.

SAGITTAL SCANS

Sagittal scans of the chest are those that cut the thorax in cephalad-caudad and anteroposterior planes (Plate III). These correspond to the usual lateral chest radiograph. In this discussion, all sagittal scans will be oriented as if an observer were on the patient's left side, so that the head is up and the spine is to the right. Sagittal scans of the entire chest are unusual but are possible when there is a large amount of pleural fluid or pulmonary congestion allowing ultrasound transmission (see Chapter 12).

Subcostal sagittal scans image the spine, descending aorta, and inferior vena cava (Figure 2–2). To the left of the spine the aorta and left crus of the diaphragm are seen together. The aorta can be identified by its arterial pulsation, celiac and superior mesenteric branches, and relatively thick walls. To the right of the spine a sagittal scan of the inferior vena cava reveals a thinner-walled structure with a typical morphologic appearance and connecting hepatic veins. The connection of the inferior vena cava to the right atrium and the eustachian valve (a constant landmark in the morphologic right atrium) can be imaged with more cephalad scanning. The course of the descending aorta behind the heart can be visualized from sagittal scans over the sternum and below it. Higher sagittal scans image the right superior vena cava, ascending aorta, and descending aorta, moving from right to left (Figure 2–3). In addition, sagittal scans from the suprasternal

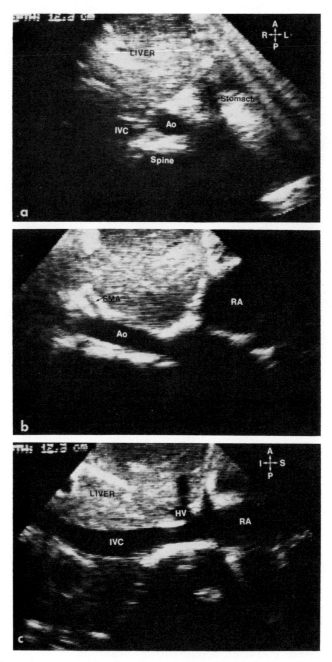

FIG. 2–2. Subcostal scans of the aorta and inferior vena cava. A transverse scan (a) shows the position of the inferior vena cava and aorta with respect to the spine. Sagittal scans (b and c) show the aorta with its superior mesenteric artery branch and the inferior vena cava with its connecting hepatic veins as it enters the right atrium.

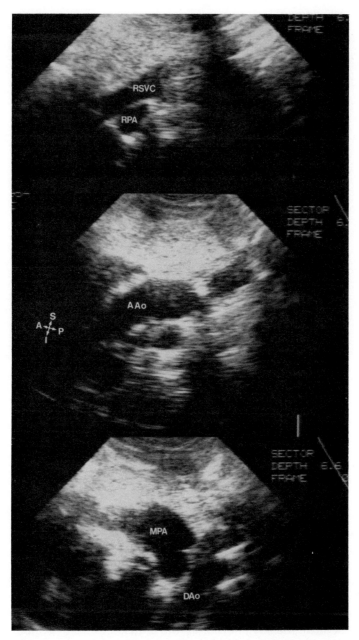

FIG. 2–3. Sagittal scans in the upper chest scanning from right to left. The right superior vena cava is seen passing immediately in front of the right pulmonary artery (upper panel). Scanning farther to the left, the ascending aorta is visualized (middle panel). Farther leftward scanning shows the main pulmonary artery and descending aorta (lower panel).

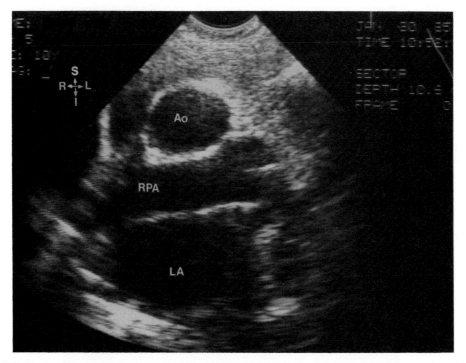

FIG. 2–4. Suprasternal coronal scan of the transverse aorta (Ao), the right pulmonary artery (RPA), and the more inferior left atrium (LA).

area in the neck can image the innominate vein, brachiocephalic vessels, and the thymus.

CORONAL SCANS

Coronal cross-sectional scans of the chest are possible from the subcostal and suprasternal ultrasound windows (Plate IV).[1] These scans resemble the corresponding anteroposterior chest radiograph, with the head up and the patient's left to the viewer's right. In this scan, the liver and diaphragm are inferior and the heart and surrounding pericardium and pleura are well visualized. From above, the pulmonary veins, systemic veins, and pulmonary arteries can be imaged (Figure 2–4). Such scans may vary slightly from tomograms using other techniques because the site of origin of the ultrasound beam is more anterior in the suprasternal or subcostal positions and therefore coronal scans may be slightly oblique anterior to posterior.

SURGERY WITHOUT ANGIOGRAPHY FOR CONGENITAL EXTRACARDIAC ABNORMALITIES

Between July 1982 and August 1985, 110 neonates, infants, and children have had corrective or palliative surgery without prior angiography at Texas Children's Hospital and Texas Heart Institute. Ultrasound imaging was used to make the definitive cardiovascular anatomic diagnosis and to examine the other aspects of the thoracic contents. Clinical information was integrated with the ultrasound findings in making a final decision in each case and the care of each patient was individualized after discussions with the parents, the pediatrician, and the surgeon. The 110 patients included 36 who were older than one year and would have had surgery without angiography in many centers prior to the advent of ultrasonography, 11 with coarctation of the aorta, five with patent ductus arteriosus, and one with vascular ring. There were 74 infants under one year of age; 50 were less than one month of age and in serious clinical difficulty either from congestive heart failure or cyanosis. This latter group included 16 with coarctation of the aorta, 12 with interrupted aortic arch, six with patent ductus arteriosus (not premature), three with total anomalous pulmonary venous connection, and four with vascular ring and stridor.

Statistical comparison of the group under one year of age (74 infants) with a similar group that had angiography, using multivariate techniques, showed that the surgical mortality rate was not significantly different in the ultrasound and angiography groups with extracardiac abnormalities. Further experience will be necessary to define the role of ultrasound imaging in the management of such infants and critically ill newborns.

REFERENCES

1. Tajik AJ, Seward JB, Hagler DJ, et al: Two-dimensional real-time ultrasonic imaging of the heart and great vessels: Technique, image orientation, structure identification, and validation. Mayo Clin Proc 53:271, 1978.
2. Silverman NH, Hunter S, Anderson RH, et al: Anatomical basis of cross sectional echocardiography. Br Heart J 50:421, 1983.
3. Silverman NH, and Snider AR: Two-Dimensional Echocardiography in Congenital Heart Disease. Norwalk, Conn: Appleton-Century-Crofts, 1982, pp 86–90.
4. Huhta JC, Smallhorn JF, and Macartney FJ: Two-dimensional echocardiographic diagnosis of situs. Br Heart J 48:97, 1982.
5. Tonkin IL, and Tonkin AD: Visceroatrial situs abnormalities: Sonographic and computed tomographic appearance. AJR 138:509, 1982.

chapter **3**

DOPPLER ULTRASOUND ASSESSMENT OF BLOOD FLOW IN THE CHEST

Doppler ultrasonography is a useful adjunct to cross-sectional ultrasonic imaging and provides an additional functional aspect to the examination of the chest. Using Doppler techniques one can assess the blood flow velocity in the imaged structure both qualitatively and quantitatively. Pulsed Doppler ultrasound functions as an intrathoracic stethoscope, which helps to answer such questions as: Is this a vascular or nonvascular structure? What is the direction of blood flow in this structure? What is the velocity of blood flow in this structure?[1,2] On the basis of some assumptions, including laminar blood flow and the cross-sectional area of flow, it is possible to estimate the stroke volume of flow by integrating the Doppler flow velocity waveform.[3]

Doppler ultrasound examination in the pediatric subject is limited by the same ultrasonic windows that allow cross-sectional echo imaging (Plate V). To obtain an adequate signal from the flow of red blood cells, the ultrasonic beam must be aligned parallel to the direction of blood flow. Cross-sectional imaging is optimal when the beam is perpendicular to the structure of interest. Therefore, a window that adequately allows echo imaging may not be adequate for Doppler signal acquisition. For example, the parasternal scan of the ascending aorta produces echo images of the aorta perpendicular to its course, but this approach for a pulsed Doppler sample volume yields poor blood flow velocity signals because the beam is not parallel to the direction of blood flow. In this case, an approach from the cardiac apex is more valuable (Figure 3–1).

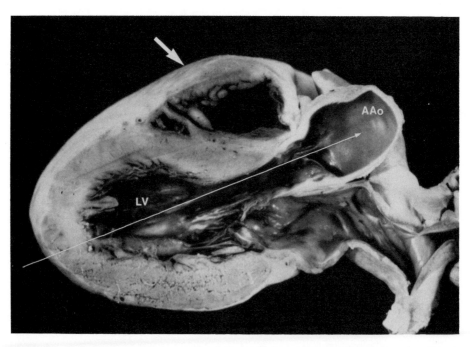

FIG. 3–1. Pathologic specimen of the left ventricle and ascending aorta showing the optimal Doppler sampling angle from the cardiac apex (long white arrow). Sampling from a parasternal scan over the chest (short white arrow) would give an unsatisfactory angle for measurement of blood flow passing from the left ventricle (LV) to the ascending aorta (AAo.)

PRINCIPLES

PULSED DOPPLER

Pulsed Doppler examination, when it is guided by cross-sectional imaging, allows placement of the sample volume at a site of interest in the ultrasound image. Extracardiac Doppler imaging utilizes principally the suprasternal, the apical, and the subcostal approaches (Plate V). Precise timing of the echoes returning after a pulse of ultrasound energy is transmitted allows gating to a given depth. The sample volume of blood flow velocity is kept as small as possible (usually 1.5 to 5.0 mm). On the cross-sectional image an indicator appears, showing the precise location of Doppler sampling in the desired structure (Plates VI and VII), and this capability is the greatest strength of pulsed Doppler examination in pediatrics. Localization of the blood flow velocity at any site in the cardiovascular system is feasible using this technique. The disadvantage of pulsed Doppler is the inability to detect velocities that fall outside the normal range for children and adults.[4] Such blood flow velocities (above twice the peak repetition frequency of sampling) limit the use of pulsed techniques for quantitative measurement or assessment at a greater depth than normal. However, good results can be obtained at shallow depths (as in aortic valve stenosis in a child) using techniques designed to extend the range of pulsed Doppler velocity measurement.[5]

CONTINUOUS WAVE DOPPLER

If interrogation of reflected Doppler shifted velocities is performed using two crystals—one for transmitting and one for receiving—the incoming signal is continuous and reflects any blood flow movement or ultrasound reflections along the entire line of the ultrasound beam. Using this technique, blood flow velocities up to and exceeding 7 m/sec can be measured.[1] The disadvantage of wholesale sampling along a line of interest is offset by the advantage of detecting very high velocities of blood flow, such as may be present in stenotic jets in congenital aortic stenosis.[6]

NORMAL FINDINGS

Aorta. Ascending aorta Doppler velocity patterns can be obtained from the apical or suprasternal approaches (Plate VIII and Figure 3–2). Normal Doppler velocity patterns in the aorta depend on the site of sampling. As pointed out by Hatle and colleagues,[1] a sampling position that is too medial in the ascending aorta will give an "abnormal" pattern because the ultrasonic beam is not centered on the major components of the systolic velocity profile. In the *ascending aorta* the pattern at the aortic valve is typical and depends on many variables, including the valve diameter, the ventricular function, the arterial impedance, and the

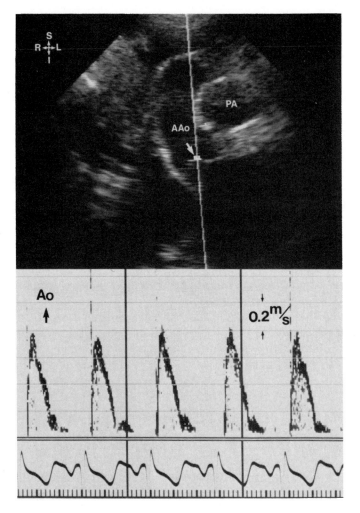

FIG. 3–2. Normal ascending aorta Doppler flow velocity from the suprasternal notch approach. The sample volume is placed near the aortic valve in the ascending aorta using a suprasternal coronal scan. The resulting Doppler velocity (bottom panel) peaks at 0.8 m/sec and has a shape suggesting an early rapid velocity during ventricular ejection.

heart rate. Higher in the ascending aorta the velocity pattern may be more turbulent, especially if the sampling site is near the wall of the aorta and not in the center. The velocity in the *descending aorta* can be obtained from the suprasternal position (Figure 3–3). Blood flow is away from the valve, and its peak velocity is attained later in the cardiac cycle.

Pulmonary Arteries. The Doppler velocity pattern in the *main pulmonary artery* is shown in Figure 3–4. In the distal *left pulmonary artery* the velocity is higher because of the smaller cross-sectional area of this vessel (Figure 3–5). This pattern is best obtained from a sagittal scan under the left clavicle. The velocity of the right pulmonary artery can be sampled from the suprasternal position. However,

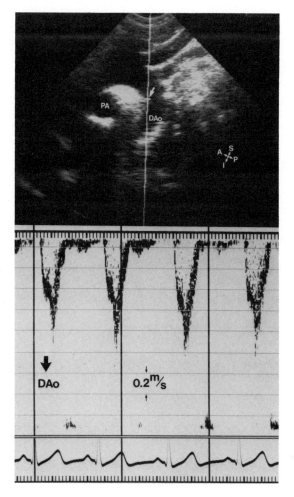

FIG. 3–3. Normal descending aorta pulsed Doppler examination. Using a suprasternal scan of the upper descending aorta (top panel), the sample volume is placed slightly distal to the left subclavian artery. The resulting flow velocity in the descending aorta (lower panel) shows an inferior direction to the systolic flow velocity, which has a peak of nearly 1.2 m/sec.

because of the orientation of the vessel, a low-angle velocity measurement is difficult.

Pulmonary Veins. Pulmonary vein flow velocities can be obtained from many positions, but we have found the suprasternal approach to be best for the lower veins, transverse scans over the chest to be best for the left upper vein, and a scan at the apex to be best for sampling the right upper pulmonary vein (see Chapter 10).

Systemic Veins. The velocity pattern in the *right superior vena cava* (SVC) is characterized by two waveforms—one during ventricular systole and one during diastole. This sampling site in the midportion of the SVC from the suprasternal approach gives lower velocities than at the entrance of the SVC into the right

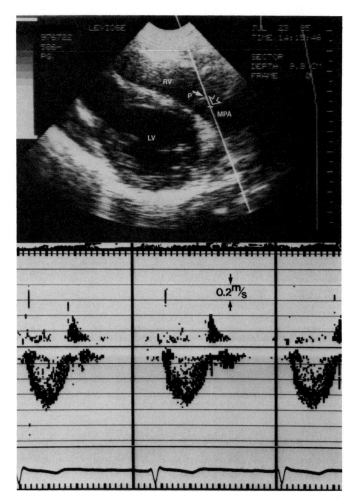

FIG. 3–4. Normal parasternal pulsed Doppler examination of the main pulmonary artery. The sample volume (open white arrow) is placed distal to the pulmonary valve (P) in the main pulmonary artery (upper panel). The resulting Doppler flow velocity has a symmetric contour in the normal pattern (lower panel) and a peak flow velocity of 0.7 m/sec.

atrium sampled from the subcostal approach (Figure 3–6). Typical flow velocity patterns in the superior vena cava are shown in Figure 3–7.

QUALITATIVE DOPPLER

One of the early uses of Doppler blood flow information was the qualitative identification of patterns and direction of blood flow. The simple identification of blood flow in a structure using pulsed Doppler examination may be important in diagnosis, e.g., in the diagnosis of chest masses (see Chapter 13). Early reports of the use of Doppler ultrasound before the development and cardiac implementation of the electronic fast Fourier transform emphasized the direction and

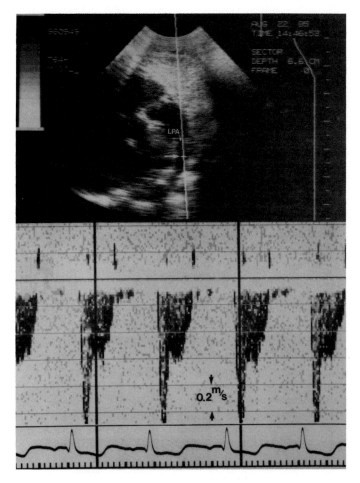

FIG. 3–5. Pulsed Doppler sampling in the left pulmonary artery from a high parasternal scan (upper panel). The sample volume is placed well distal to the origin of the left pulmonary artery (LPA), near the location where it crosses the descending aorta. The pulsed Doppler velocity pattern (lower panel) shows a velocity higher than in the main pulmonary artery because of the smaller size of the left pulmonary artery.

pattern of blood flow velocity in some congenital abnormalities. With modern methods of instantaneous velocity measurement, qualitative observations are much more accurate. For example, right-to-left reversal of flow (which suggests pulmonary hypertension) in a patient with ductus arteriosus can be detected (Figure 3–8). Pulsed Doppler has the advantage of "scanning" from one flow velocity to another, providing results much the same as a catheter pullback during cardiac catheterization (Figure 3–9).

Color flow mapping of Dopper flow velocities can be superimposed on the cross-sectional image. There are many examples of the qualitative use of this technology at the present time.[7] Detection of shunts and the measurement of the angle of stenotic jets has already found application in clinical cardiology. The promise of quantitation of valvar regurgitation has expanded the use of this technique. Early experience in our center has shown color flow mapping to be

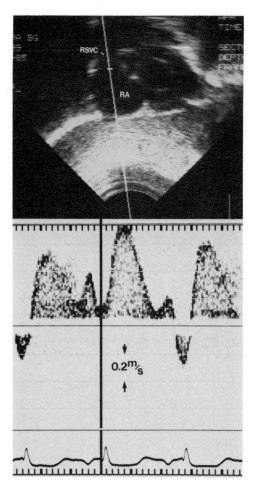

FIG. 3–6. Normal pulsed Doppler pattern in the superior vena cava obtained from the subcostal approach. The pulsed Doppler sample volume is placed in the orifice of the superior vena cava where it enters the right atrium. The resulting pulsed Doppler waveform in this newborn baby shows normal superior vena caval velocities of nearly 0.8 m/sec, with marked variations related to respiration and the cardiac cycle.

superior to imaging/Doppler in the detection of multiple defects of the ventricular septum.[8]

QUANTITATIVE DOPPLER

CARDIAC OUTPUT MEASUREMENT

Doppler quantitation of blood flow is based on the principle that the mean velocity of red blood cells passing any point expressed in centimeters per second times the cross-sectional area at that point (centimeters squared) equals the flow in cubic centimeters (cc) per second (flow = mean velocity × area). Obtaining

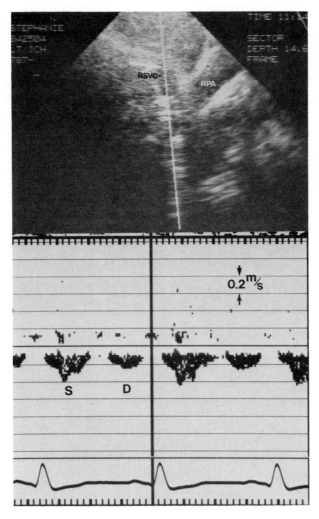

FIG. 3–7. Right superior vena caval (RSVC) blood flow velocity pattern obtained from the suprasternal notch approach. The sample volume is placed in the high right superior vena cava, and the resulting flow velocity pattern (lower panel) shows a systolic (S) and a diastolic component (D) to inferiorly oriented caval blood flow.

this information noninvasively requires several assumptions, including a Doppler sampling location that allows sampling precisely perpendicular to the cross-sectional area of the vessel or valve, a knowledge of the exact area, and a single, laminar flow velocity value at each instant during the cardiac cycle.

Little information is available about possible correlation of Doppler information with aortic blood flow in children measured simultaneously by another method. Preliminary data in the intensive care unit of Texas Children's Hospital collected by Morrow and Murphy using continuous wave Doppler techniques showed a good correlation between Doppler and thermodilution cardiac outputs (Figure 3–10). Of more importance for the patient is the possibility of serial measurements of stroke volume before and after an intervention designed to improve

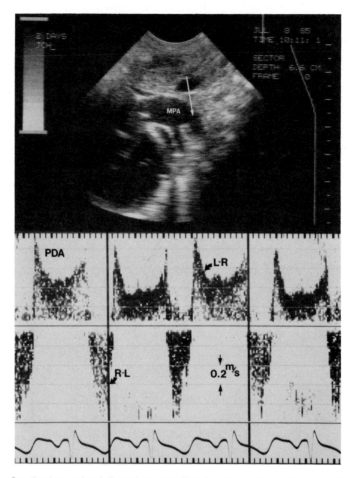

FIG. 3–8. Qualitative pulsed Doppler sampling in the ductus arteriosus of a 2-day-old infant. Note the right-to-left ductal shunting occurring late in systole (R-L). There appeared to be variations in the magnitude of left-to-right (L-R) shunting based on respiratory changes.

the cardiac output. Early results suggest that this method is useful in spite of changes in blood pressure, heart rate, and systemic vascular resistance.

PULMONARY/SYSTEMIC FLOW RATIO MEASUREMENTS

The ratio of the pulmonary to the systemic flow in a lesion that causes a left-to-right shunt can be estimated by the use of Doppler measurement of the time-velocity integral and the measurement of the valve anuli by cross-sectional imaging (Figure 3–11).[3,9] Significant limitations exist in this technique related to the accurate measurement of the cross-sectional area of the anuli, but we find it useful to estimate the shunt magnitude in the postoperative patient and in the premature infant.

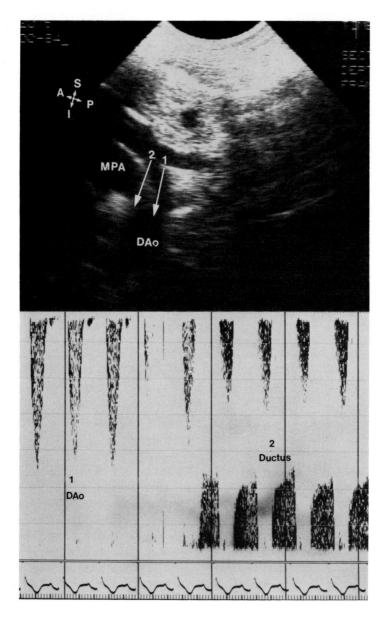

FIG. 3–9. Suprasternal scan of the main pulmonary artery and descending aorta. The pulsed Doppler sample volume was moved from the descending aorta (1) into the region of the ductus arteriosus (2) (upper panel). The resulting Doppler velocity pattern in the descending aorta (1) and bidirectional ductal shunting in the ductus arteriosus (2) are shown (lower panel).

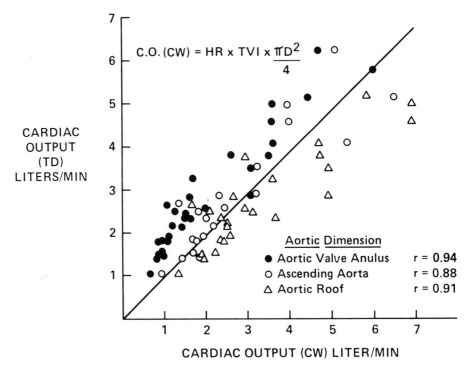

FIG. 3–10. Data from continuous wave Doppler measurements of cardiac output showing the correlation with thermal dilution cardiac outputs. Note that the optimal values are obtained by utilizing the aortic valve anulus for calculation of the cross-sectional area of blood flow.

PRESSURE GRADIENT MEASUREMENT

Quantitation of pressure gradients using the modified Bernoulli equation allows estimation of the minimum gradient across a stenosis (Figure 3–12). The accuracy of such a measurement depends on the angle of the Doppler sampling. If the angle is 20 degrees or less, little error is introduced into the calculation. The gradient in millimeters of mercury (mm Hg) is equal to the Doppler peak blood flow velocity squared times four. This modification of the Bernoulli equation assumes that (1) the kinetic energy of the blood well downstream to the obstruction is negligible, and (2) the energy of acceleration of blood during systole can be ignored.

$$\text{Gradient (mm Hg)} = 4(v_1^2 - v_2^2) \qquad (1)$$

where v_1 is the velocity proximal to the obstruction and v_2 is the velocity distal. If $v_2 \ll v_1$, then for clinical use:

$$\text{Gradient (mm Hg)} = 4(v_1^2)* \qquad (2)$$

---

*A detailed derivation of this equation can be found in Chapter 8 of Goldberg SJ, Allen HD, Marx GR, and Flinn CJ: Doppler Echocardiography. Philadelphia, Lea & Febiger, 1985.

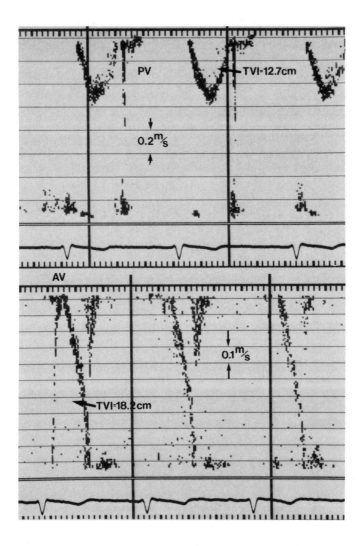

FIG. 3–11. Parasternal pulmonary valve blood flow velocity (upper panel) and suprasternal ascending aorta flow velocity (lower panel) in a 5-year-old girl, following atrial septal defect repair. Calculations of Qp/Qs showed it to be 0.9, which is within the range of normal; this girl had no residual left-to-right shunt. TVI = the time velocity integral that is the area under the Doppler tracing.

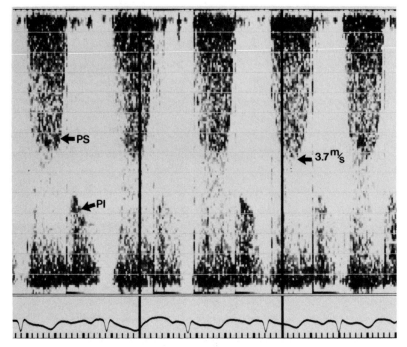

FIG. 3–12. Quantitative Doppler assessment of the severity of pulmonary stenosis in a patient following repair of tetralogy of Fallot. Note the systolic jet at approximately 3.7 m/sec, corresponding to moderate pulmonary stenosis. There was mild pulmonary insufficiency (PI) in the opposite direction.

Use of this principle to calculate the severity of an obstruction in the ascending aorta is illustrated in Figure 5–7.

REFERENCES

1. Hatle L, and Angelsen B: Doppler Ultrasound in Cardiology. Physical Principles and Clinical Applications. Philadelphia, Lea & Febiger, 1982, p. 89.
2. Goldberg SJ, Allen HD, Marx GR, and Flinn CJ: Doppler Echocardiography. Philadelphia, Lea & Febiger, 1985.
3. Sanders SP, Yeager S, and Williams RG: Measurement of systemic and pulmonary blood flow and QP/QS ratio using Doppler and two-dimensional echocardiography. Am J Cardiol 51:952, 1983.
4. Grenadier E, Oliveira-Lima C, Allen HD, et al: Normal intracardiac and great vessel Doppler flow velocities in infants and children. J Am Coll Cardiol 4:343, 1984.
5. Stevenson JG, and Kawabori I: Noninvasive determination of pressure gradients in children: Two methods employing pulsed Doppler echocardiography. J Am Coll Cardiol 3:179, 1984.
6. Hatle L: Noninvasive assessment and differentiation of left ventricular outflow obstruction with Doppler ultrasound. Circulation 64:381, 1981.
7. Sahn DJ: Real-time two-dimensional Doppler echocardiographic flow mapping. (Review.) Circulation 71:849, 1985.
8. Ludomirsky A, Vick GW, Morrow WR, et al: Two-dimensional color flow mapping for detection of multiple/muscular ventricular septal defects. Presented at the AHA, Washington, D.C., Nov. 1985.
9. Vargas-Barron J, Sahn DJ, Valdes-Cruz LM, et al.: Clinical utility of two-dimensional Doppler echocardiographic techniques for estimating pulmonary to systemic blood flow ratios in children with left to right shunting atrial septal defect, ventricular septal defect or patent ductus arteriosus. J Am Coll Cardiol 3:169, 1984.

chapter 4

THYMUS, TRACHEA,
AND ESOPHAGUS

Three midline structures that have importance in pediatric diagnosis of abnormalities of the thorax are the thymus, the trachea, and the esophagus (Plates IX and X). Each may be important in the assessment of extracardiac congenital or acquired lung or heart disease.

THYMUS

NORMAL

The normal thymus in a newborn infant is a relatively large structure lying anterior to the heart in the midline in a retrosternal, extrapleural position. In the newborn, the thymus is a large structure and may be so large as to suggest cardiomegaly. Ultrasound imaging of the thymus is feasible from the suprasternal approach in most children. It appears as an irregular anterior mass with a homogeneous density that readily transmits ultrasound energy (Figure 4–1). Overlying the innominate vein (see Chapter 11), the thymus lacks a discrete capsule so that it tends to fuse with the surrounding structures. With increasing age after birth, significant involution of the thymus occurs, but this structure remains an asset to ultrasound imaging throughout infancy.

ABNORMAL

The most common abnormality of the thymus in the infant is hypoplasia or aplasia, part of the spectrum of DiGeorge's syndrome and often associated with

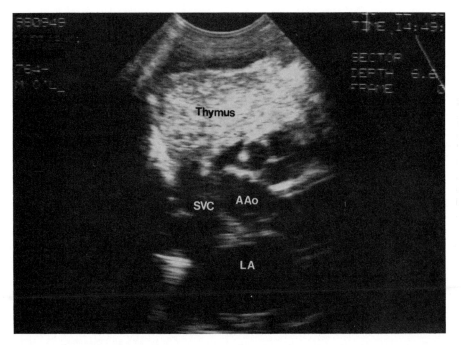

FIG. 4–1. Suprasternal notch ultrasonic imaging of the normal thymus in a newborn baby. Note the homogeneous echo density and transmission capabilities of this structure.

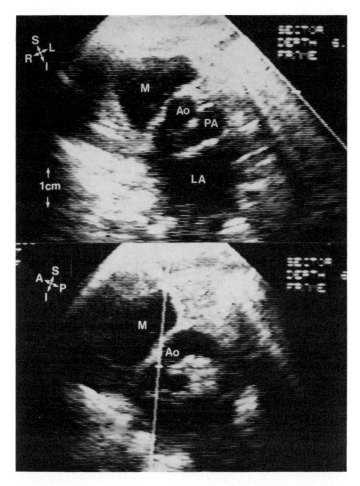

FIG. 4–2. Suprasternal scanning of a dilated thoracic duct in a newborn infant with persistent chylothorax. The mass (M) was superior to the aorta and in the region of the thymus. Such a mass could not be differentiated from a cystic hygroma or a thymoma.

underdevelopment of the parathyroid glands and hypocalcemia. Some forms of congenital heart disease are associated with DiGeorge's syndrome, including tetralogy of Fallot with right aortic arch, interrupted aortic arch, pulmonary atresia with ventricular septal defect, and truncus arteriosus.[1] In a recent review of echocardiographic findings in DiGeorge's syndrome at Texas Children's Hospital, there was no diagnostic marker of aplasia of the thymus. The well-known adage that "absence of evidence is not evidence of absence" applies here; however, the presence of echolucency above the aortic arch and generalized poor suprasternal ultrasound penetration are highly suggestive of thymic aplasia in the newborn infant.

Thymoma appears as an echo-free cystic mass in the location of the normal thymus. A dilated thoracic duct or cystic hygroma may cause a mass in an identical location (Figures 4–2 and 4–3). The ultrasonic diagnosis of cystic hygroma in the fetus is now feasible. Such masses may grow to a large size, causing symptoms resulting from compression of other thoracic structures.[2]

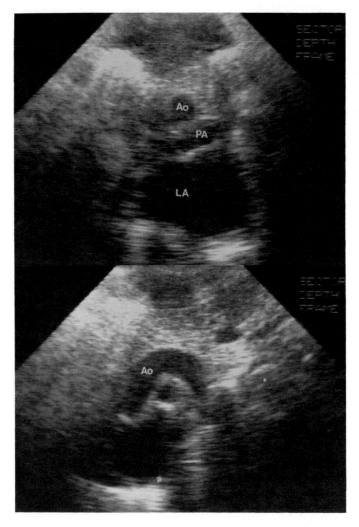

FIG. 4–3. Scan of the same infant as in Figure 4–2 two weeks later showing resolution of the mass following fat-free feedings. Obstruction of the thoracic duct is suggested as the cause of the mass.

TRACHEA

The trachea is a cartilaginous tube that transmits air to and from the lungs. Because the trachea contains air, it is not well visualized by ultrasound imaging. The left bronchus can be visualized during scanning of the aortic arch in some patients (see Chapter 6). The trachea and the esophagus run together in the midline and both can be used as markers in the determination of the side of the aortic arch. A significant shift of the trachea to one side of the chest may be a clue to atelectasis on the side of the shift or a mass in the contralateral chest.

Although adequate imaging of the trachea is not possible in most patients because it is an air-filled structure, ultrasonography may be a useful tool in the

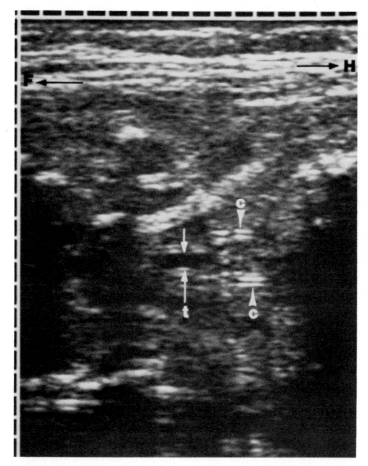

FIG. 4–4. Fetal echocardiogram of the fetal trachea (t) and carotid arteries (c). (Used by permission of Dr. C. Cooper. Reprinted from J. Ultrasound Med., *4*:343, 1985.) H = head, F = feet.

evaluation of the trachea in the fetus.[3] In a study by Cooper and coworkers,[3] the fetal trachea was adequately imaged lying between the two carotid arteries (Figures 4–4 and 4–5) in 47 of 50 human fetuses studied prospectively and ranged in size from 2 to 4 mm (mean size 2.6 mm). Tracheal fluid flow in the human fetal trachea has been studied by Doppler ultrasound.[4]

ESOPHAGUS

The esophagus is a muscular tube, and the passage of food and liquid during swallowing can be observed by ultrasonic imaging even though the esophageal wall itself cannot be well imaged. The esophagus usually contains a mixture of liquid and air whose movement can be visualized by ultrasound imaging (Figure 4–6). Such spontaneous contrast or that following feeding the patient a liquid is useful for identification of the midline in a manner similar to that for the

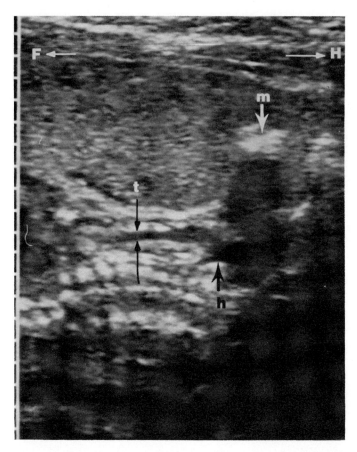

FIG. 4–5. Ultrasonic imaging of the hypopharynx and the trachea in a fetus. The mouth (m) and hypopharynx at the origin of the esophagus (h) are well visualized, as is the trachea (t). (Used by permission of Dr. C. Cooper. Reprinted from J. Ultrasound Med., 4:343, 1985.) H = head, F = feet.

trachea. This method of marking the midline is reliable and useful in the determination of the side of the aortic arch (see Chapter 6).[5] Little data are available concerning the use of ultrasound in this way in the newborn, but it is possible to see the ultrasonic reflections from esophageal content, and such a method may be useful in the diagnosis of gastroesophageal reflux.

In the fetus, the esophagus is probably collapsed in its resting state.[3] The diagnosis of esophageal atresia has been made in the human fetus by ultrasound imaging.[6–8] The distended proximal esophageal pouch is visible on the antenatal sonogram as a clue to this diagnosis. In the neonate the absence of normal esophageal contrast passing to the stomach may indicate the presence of a congenital tracheal abnormality in association with esophageal atresia. The surgical approach to esophageal atresia with a tracheoesophageal fistula is dependent on knowledge of the side of the descending aorta. Such a decision can be made using ultrasound without other studies.

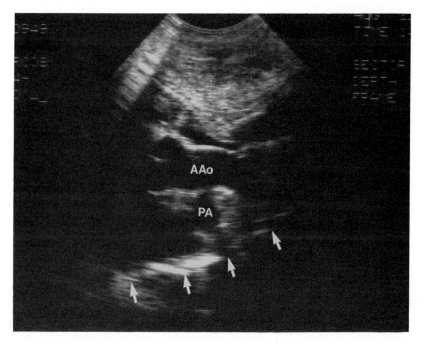

FIG. 4–6. Sagittal scanning of the esophagus during swallowing showing the ultrasonic reflections from liquid in the esophagus (white arrows). This technique is used in conjunction with imaging of the spine and trachea to identify the midline for determination of the side of the aortic arch.

REFERENCES

1. Freedom RM, Rosen FS, and Nadas AS: Congenital cardiovascular disease and anomalies of the third and fourth laryngeal pouch. Circulation 46:165, 1972.
2. Grosfeld JL, Weber TR, and Vane DW: One-stage resection for massive cervicomediastinal hygroma. Surgery 92:693, 1982.
3. Cooper C, Mahony BS, Bowie JD, et al: Ultrasound evaluation of the normal fetal upper airway and esophagus. J Ultrasound Med 4:343, 1985.
4. Utsu M, Sakakibara S, Ishida T, et al: Dynamics of tracheal fluid flow in the human fetus, studied with pulsed Doppler ultrasound. Acta Obstet Gynecol Jpn 35:2017, 1983.
5. Huhta JC, Gutgesell HP, Latson LA, and Huffines FD: Two-dimensional echocardiographic assessment of the aorta in infants and children with congenital heart disease. Circulation 70:417, 1984.
6. Farrant P: The antenatal diagnosis of oesophageal atresia by ultrasound. Br J Radiol 53:1202, 1980.
7. Pretorius DH, Meier PR, and Johnson ML: Diagnosis of esophageal atresia in utero. J Ultrasound Med 2:475, 1983.
8. Eyheremendy E, and Pfister M: Antenatal real-time diagnosis of esophageal atresias. J Clin Ultrasound 11:395, 1983.

chapter **5**

ASCENDING AORTA

The ascending aorta begins from a left posteroinferior position at the aortic valve and continues to a right anterosuperior position at the transverse arch. Arising from the normal left ventricle, the plane of the ascending aorta moves from transverse to sagittal, so that it changes direction as it ascends the chest.

NORMAL

Because the ascending aorta is a tubular structure, a single tomographic plane cannot describe it completely. Illustrated views of the ascending aorta commonly fail to image its intrapericardial aspect near the aortic valve. Therefore, the ascending aorta must be scanned from a suprasternal or sternal approach in order to examine the inferior portion (Plate XI) and from a suprasternal approach to examine the more superior aspect (Plate XII). With counterclockwise rotation of the transducer in the suprasternal notch, one may scan from one projection to the other (Figure 5–1).

DILATION

Enlargement of the ascending aorta may result from increased flow through it for several reasons, including (1) patent ductus arteriosus or aortic regurgitation, (2) turbulence above an area of outflow tract obstruction, such as aortic valve stenosis,[2] or (3) weakening of the vessel wall, as occurs in patients with Marfan's disease. The appearance of dilation of the ascending aorta may be a clue to the cause. In dilation resulting from increased flow there is uniform, tubular enlargement of this structure. One of the most common causes of this appearance is transposition of the great arteries (Figure 5–2).

The dilation seen downstream from a stenosis is usually localized at the impact site of the jet (Figure 5–3). Quantitation of the degree of poststenotic dilation may aid diagnosis of critical aortic stenosis (Figure 5–4). Dramatic ascending aortic dilation may result from a congenital abnormality called left ventricular to aortic tunnel. Massive aortic to left ventricular regurgitation greatly increases the amount of blood pumped into the ascending aorta each systole, resulting in its enlargement (Figure 5–5).

HYPOPLASIA

Decreased size of the ascending aorta is usually associated with decreased aortic flow. For example, in neonates with interrupted aortic arch the ascending aorta supplies only a portion of the upper body. In this abnormality the aortic hypoplasia may be a limiting factor in normal cardiac output following surgical correction. The most severe hypoplasia of the ascending aorta occurs in association with hypoplastic left-sided heart syndrome (Figure 5–6A). Here the flow velocity is retrograde from normal, and the ascending aorta is supplying only the coronary arteries (Figure 5–6B).

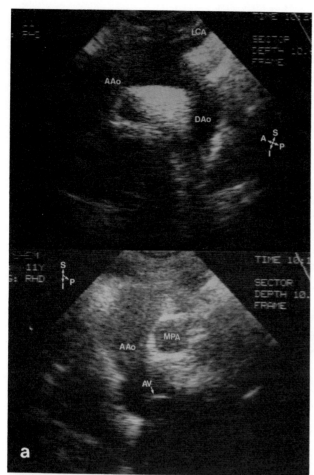

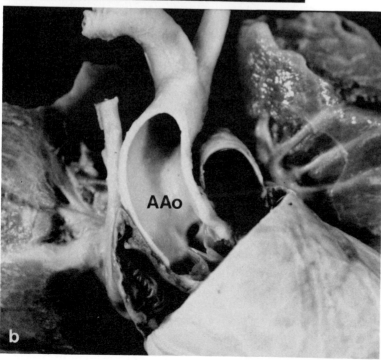

FIG. 5–1. (a) A normal ascending aorta illustrating the supravalvar region (upper panel) and the more superior portion of the ascending aorta (lower panel). Compare with Plates XI and XII. (b) Pathologic specimen cut to illustrate the normal plane of the ascending aorta.

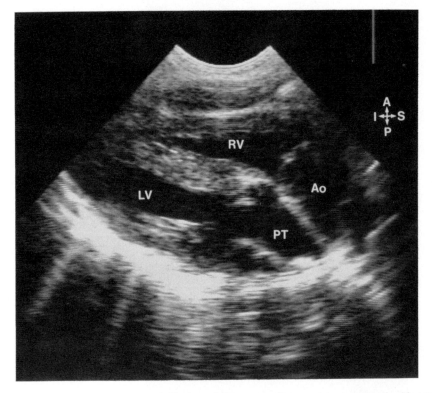

FIG. 5–2. Ultrasound imaging of dilation of the ascending aorta associated with transposition of the great arteries. Note the aorta (Ao) from the right ventricle (RV) and the pulmonary trunk (PT) from the left ventricle (LV).

OBSTRUCTION

Supravalvar aortic stenosis is the most common cause of obstruction of the ascending aorta in children. This discrete narrowing is often intimately associated with the aortic valve cusps (Figure 5–7). The resultant increase in ascending aortic blood flow velocity can be measured by Doppler ultrasound in order to assess the severity of the obstruction (see Chapter 3).[3]

Ascending aortic narrowing may result from aortic cannulation at the time of cardiac surgery but rarely is this a significant factor.

AORTOPULMONARY COMMUNICATIONS

Congenital communications between the ascending aorta and the pulmonary circulation are rare and few in number. When there is a defect in septation of the embryonic truncus, an aortopulmonary (AP) window may result. The communication is usually large (Figure 5–8), allowing a large left-to-right shunt and resulting in symptoms of congestive heart failure early in infancy. Because this defect occurs in the area near the pericardial reflection, it must be specifically

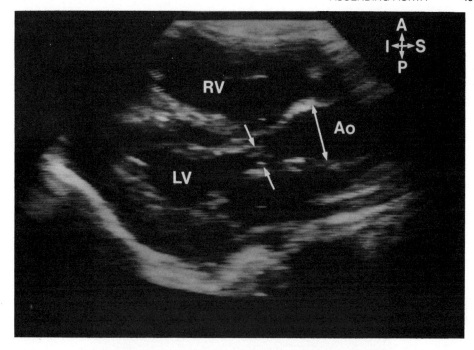

FIG. 5–3. Ultrasound imaging of poststenotic dilation of the ascending aorta in a neonate with aortic valve stenosis. (From Circulation *70*:438, 1984.)

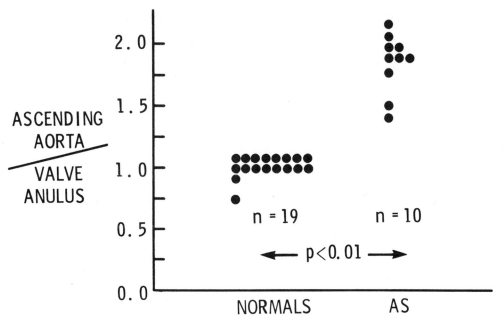

FIG. 5–4. Quantitative measurements from ultrasonic examination of the aorta, ascending aorta, and the aortic valve anulus in normal neonates and those with aortic valve stenosis. A ratio greater than 1.4 was strongly suggestive of poststenotic dilation secondary to aortic valve stenosis. (From Circulation *70*:438, 1984.)

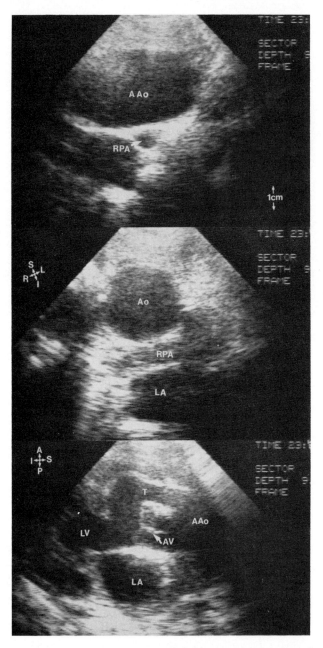

FIG. 5–5. Ultrasound imaging of a patient with left ventricular to ascending aorta tunnel with marked dilation of the ascending aorta (AAo). This can be seen in transverse scans of the ascending aorta (upper panel) and in coronal cross-sections of this dilated structure (middle panel). Aortic dilation in this case was caused by marked aortic regurgitation due to increased stroke volume into the ascending aorta from the tunnel (T), bypassing the aortic valve (AV) (lower panel).

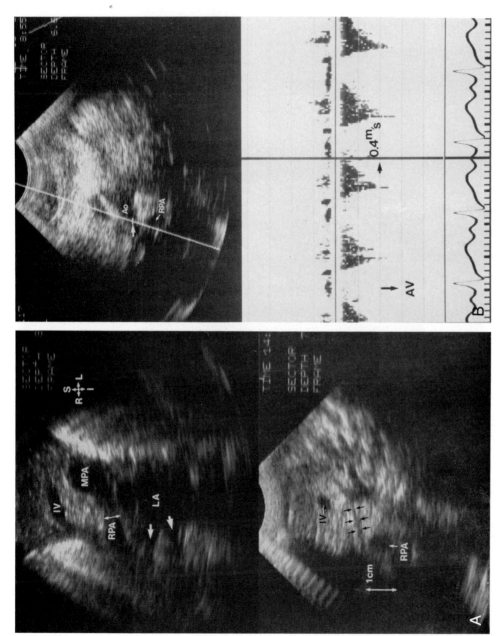

FIG. 5–6. (A) Ultrasound imaging of hypoplasia of the ascending aorta in a patient with hypoplastic left-sided heart syndrome. The ascending aorta (black arrows) measured 2 mm in diameter in this neonate (lower panel). White arrows show normal right pulmonary veins. (B) Reversed ascending aortic flow velocity caused by aortic atresia. Arrows indicate the site of pulsed Doppler sampling. AV = the direction of the aortic valve.

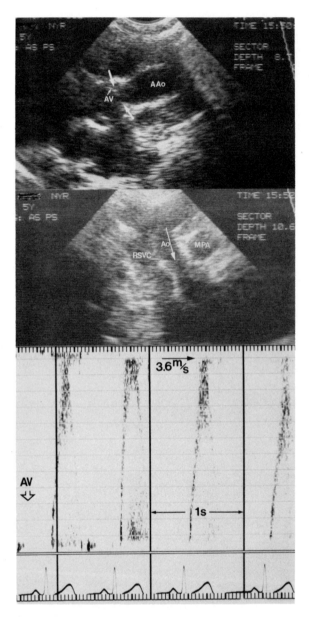

FIG. 5–7. Supravalvar aortic stenosis imaged by ultrasonography from the parasternal (upper panel) and suprasternal (middle panel) approaches. The pulsed Doppler sampling volume was placed immediately above the obstruction and measured a 3.6 m/sec left ventricle to aortic blood velocity, confirming the presence of moderately severe obstruction (lower panel).

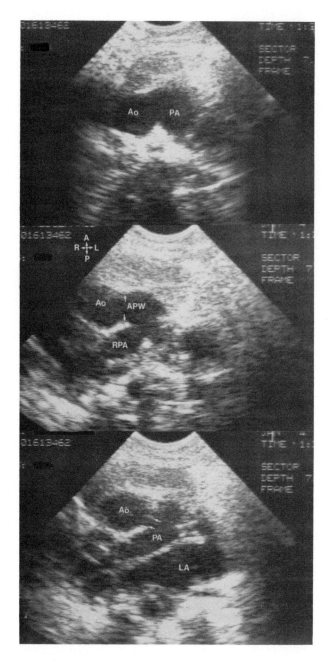

FIG. 5–8. Ultrasound parasternal imaging of aortopulmonary window (APW). Scanning more anteriorly, large intercommunication between the ascending aorta and the main pulmonary artery is seen (white arrows in lower panel).

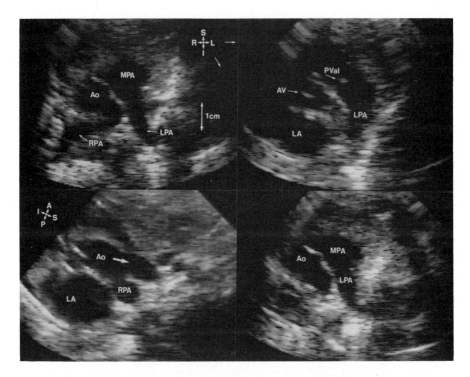

FIG. 5–9. Ultrasound scanning of anomalous origin of the right pulmonary artery from the ascending aorta. The presence of two semilunar valves distinguishes this condition from truncus arteriosus; a lack of normal pulmonary artery continuity separates this condition from that of AP window. (Reprinted with permission from the American College of Cardiology. J Am Coll Cardiol 4:351, 1984.)

excluded during each examination.[4] The Doppler pattern of AP window is similar for all AP communications affecting the ascending aorta, with diastolic reversal of blood flow velocity. This defect must be differentiated from that of origin of the right pulmonary artery from the ascending aorta.[5] In the latter condition, there are two semilunar valves, as in AP window; however the right pulmonary artery is not in continuity with the left (Figure 5–9). AP window may coexist with other defects, and one recent example of this at Texas Children's Hospital was AP window with interrupted aortic arch (Figure 5–10).

In truncus arteriosus both pulmonary arteries originate from the common truncal root. There may be a common origin, a nearly common origin, or a separate origin of the pulmonary arteries (Figure 5–11).

A rare abnormality of the ascending aorta is aortico-left ventricular tunnel. In this lesion, there is an anomalous channel from the ascending aorta to the left ventricle, bypassing the aortic valve. In this unusual cause of aortic insufficiency, Doppler sampling in the tunnel shows retrograde flow velocity.[6]

ACQUIRED ABNORMALITIES

Acquired abnormalities of the ascending aorta in children are usually post-surgical. Aneurysms of the ascending aorta may be caused by a weakened aortic

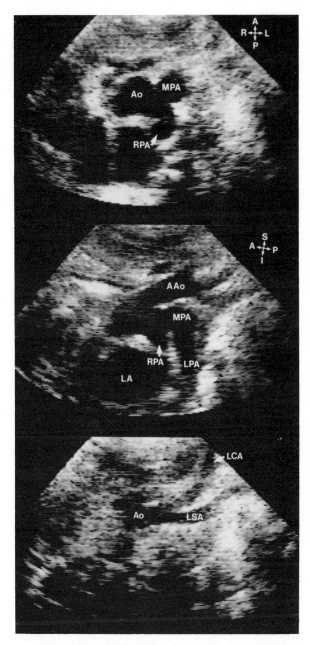

FIG. 5–10. Ultrasound imaging of AP window in combination wth interrupted aortic arch between the left subclavian artery and descending aorta. Parasternal (upper panel) and suprasternal scans (middle and lower panels) show the large aorto-pulmonary communication and the lack of aortic continuity. (Reprinted with permission from the American College of Cardiology. J Am Coll Cardiol 4:351, 1984.)

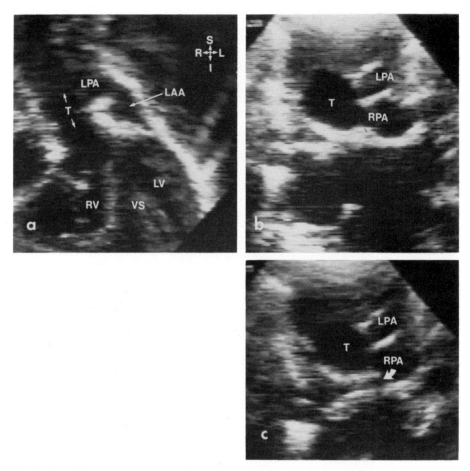

FIG. 5–11. Ultrasound imaging of truncus arteriosus and the origin of the pulmonary arteries from the ascending aorta. (a) Subcostal scan showing the overriding truncus (T) and the possible overlap of the left pulmonary artery (LPA) and the left atrial appendage (LAA). (b) and (c) Suprasternal scans of the unusual course of the right pulmonary artery (RPA) in truncus.

wall. A large aneurysm of the ascending aorta was a late surgical complication in a six-year-old boy at the site of a previous aorta to right pulmonary artery Goretex® anastomosis. This aneurysm presented as a right lung mass and was found to be vascular after Doppler sampling near its origin (see Chapter 13).

Patients with Marfan's disease may manifest aortic root dilation in childhood (Figure 5–12). The aortic dilation associated with this syndrome may allow in utero diagnosis.[7,8] A child with evidence of dilated aortic sinuses should have careful intracardiac evaluation for mitral valve prolapse, and ultrasonography provides an excellent means to follow the enlargement of the aorta and evaluate for possible dissection of the aortic wall.[9]

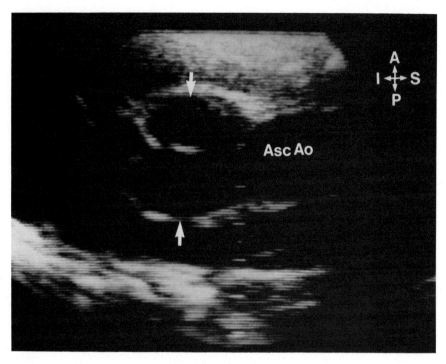

FIG. 5–12. Ultrasound imaging of the ascending aortic (AscAo) dilation and the aortic sinus dilation (white arrows) seen in Marfan's syndrome.

REFERENCES

1. Huhta JC, Latson LA, Gutgesell HP, et al: Echocardiography in the diagnosis and management of symptomatic aortic valve stenosis in infants. Circulation 70:438, 1984.
2. Come PC, Fortuin NJ, White RI Jr, and McKusick VA: Echocardiographic assessment of cardiovascular abnormalities in the Marfan syndrome. Comparison with clinical findings and with roentgenographic estimation of aortic root size. Am J Med 74:465, 1983.
3. Kosturakis D, Allen HD, Goldberg SJ, et al: Noninvasive quantification of stenotic semilunar valve areas by Doppler echocardiography. J Am Coll Cardiol 3:1256, 1984.
4. Rice MJ, Seward JB, Hagler DJ, et al: Visualization of aortopulmonary window by two-dimensional echocardiography. Mayo Clin Proc 57:482, 1982.
5. King D, Huhta JC, Gutgesell HP, and Ott DA: Two-dimensional echocardiographic diagnosis of anomalous origin of the right pulmonary artery from the aorta: Differentiation from aortopulmonary window. J Am Coll Cardiol 4:351, 1984.
6. Bash SE, Huhta JC, Nihill MR, et al: Aortico-left ventricular tunnel with ventricular septal defect: Two-dimensional/Doppler echocardiographic diagnosis. J Am Coll Cardiol 5:757, 1985.
7. Lababidi Z, and Monzon C: Early cardiac manifestations of Marfan's syndrome in the newborn. Am Heart J 102:943, 1981.
8. Koenigsberg M, Factor S, Cho S, et al.: Fetal Marfan syndrome: Prenatal ultrasound diagnosis with pathological confirmation of skeletal and aortic lesions. Prenat Diagn 1:241, 1981.
9. Mattleman S, Panidis I, Kotler MN, et al: Dissecting aneurysm in a patient with Marfan's syndrome: Recognition of extensive involvement of the aorta by two-dimensional echocardiography. JCU 12:219, 1984.

chapter **6**

AORTIC ARCH

A broad spectrum of abnormalities may affect the aortic arch. A logical analysis of the presumed embryology of such abnormalities has been proposed.[1] A segmental approach to the aortic arch and its branches is useful in diagnosis and can be accomplished by cross-sectional ultrasonography.[2,3]

NORMAL

A complete description of the arch includes (1) the side of the aortic arch, (2) the origin and course of the carotid and subclavian arteries, and (3) the side, size, and course of the upper descending aorta. Ultrasound scans for analysis of the arch are obtained predominantly from the suprasternal notch and high sternal approaches (Plates XIII and XIV).

SIDE OF THE ARCH

Cross-sectional ultrasound diagnosis of the side of the aortic arch has been described using several techniques. As with much of noninvasive study, it is preferable to combine several methods to obtain an accurate answer in every patient. Identifying the position of the transducer during visualization of the upper descending aorta is the most straightforward approach.[4] In cases with normal orientation of the ascending and descending aorta, the experienced examiner can be quite certain of the side of the arch with this alone. However, in patients with complex congenital heart disease or pulmonary defect, midline displacement errors can occur. With a midline marker such as the trachea or esophagus, the side of the transverse aortic arch can be diagnosed with confidence. This is possible either by direct visualization of the trachea, which is relatively reflective of ultrasonic waves, or by visualization of the esophagus by imaging swallowed liquid in sagittal scans and then locating the transverse aorta.[3] We have found that administration of a very small amount of carbonated liquid allows easy, rapid recognition of the esophagus (see Chapter 4).

AORTIC ARCH BRANCHING

The two carotid and two subclavian arterial branches of the aortic arch should be imaged in every ultrasound examination of the chest. Normally, the innominate artery arises from the side opposite the aortic arch. From the suprasternal approach, with a normal left aortic arch and normal brachiocephalic branching, the transducer is aimed toward the right shoulder, scanning the transverse aorta and the carotid and subclavian branches of the innominate artery (Figure 6–1). In patients with anomalous origin of the subclavian artery (see further on), this method is not confirmatory of the side of the arch. It may, however, be useful in situations such as esophageal atresia, in which the side of the arch is important, there usually is normal branching, and the usual midline marker is not available.

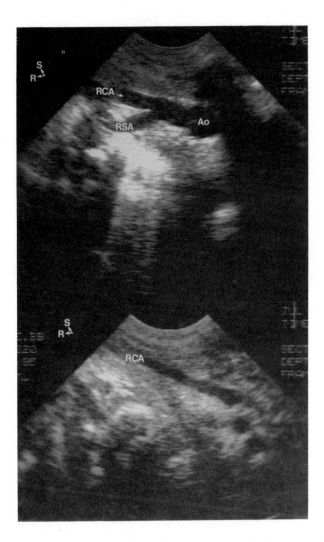

FIG. 6–1. Ultrasound scan of the normal right innominate artery (upper panel). The normal branching of the right carotid artery (RCA) and right subclavian artery (RSA) can be seen. This identifies a left aortic arch with normal branching (compare with Plate XIII). With an anomalous right subclavian artery, only the right carotid branch is seen (lower panel).

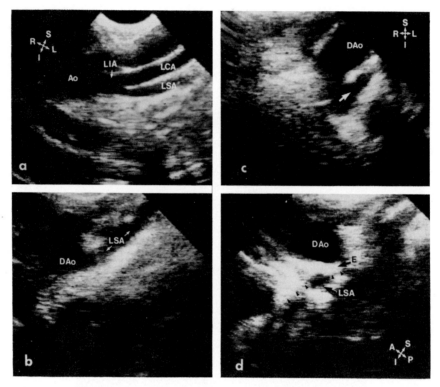

FIG. 6–2. Ultrasound scan from the suprasternal notch of a patient with right aortic arch and mirror image branching. (a) The scan toward the left shoulder shows the left innominate artery (LIA) branching into the left carotid artery (LCA) and left subclavian artery (LSA). In (b), (c), and (d), with a right arch and an anomalous left subclavian artery, the retroesophageal course can be imaged. Visualization of the esophagus (E) during swallowing confirms the abnormal LSA course (d). (From Circulation 70:417, 1984.)

ABNORMALITIES

The size of the brachiocephalic branches is sometimes useful as a clue to diagnosis. For example, in patients with congestive heart failure caused by a peripheral arteriovenous fistula, the artery supplying the fistula will be dilated. In children with cerebral arteriovenous fistula, the carotid arteries are increased in size because of the increased flow through them. In coarctation of the aorta collateral arteries may arise from the aortic arch branches, resulting in enlargement. Diastolic runoff indicating the presence of significant flow via arch vessel collaterals can be assessed by Doppler sampling.

RIGHT AORTIC ARCH

Right aortic arch with normal or mirror image branching is most commonly associated with a congenital cardiac abnormality. In patients with a right aortic arch and mirror-image branching, the innominate, left carotid, and subclavian

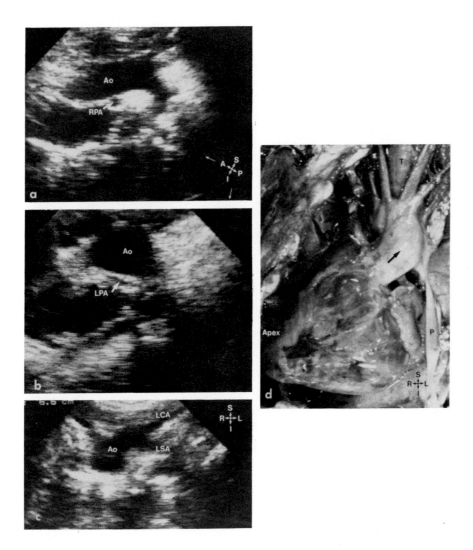

FIG. 6–3. An infant with dextrocardia and the course of the ascending aorta toward the left with a right aortic arch and mirror image branching. The descending aorta was to the right of the spine (a) and (b). The normal left innominate artery is seen in (c), with its normal branches to the left. (d) Autopsy in the same infant showing the abnormal direction of the ascending aorta (black arrow). P = pericardium.

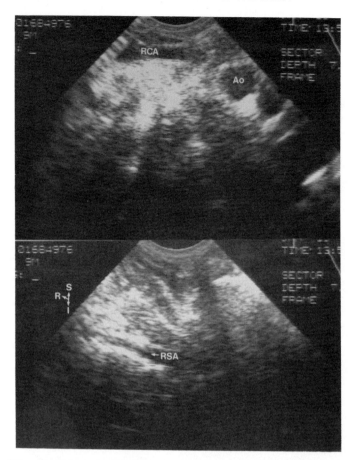

FIG. 6–4. Ultrasound images showing abnormal aortic arch branching with a left aortic arch. The upper panel shows the innominate artery consisting of only the right carotid artery. This lack of normal arch branching in the presence of a left aortic arch is highly suggestive of anomalous right subclavian artery with left aortic arch and this is confirmed with more posterior scanning (lower panel).

artery branches are seen by aiming the transducer toward the left shoulder (Figure 6–2). In sagittal scans of the main and left pulmonary arteries, the normal visualization of the descending aorta is lacking. During suprasternal scanning it is important to avoid the error of excessive counter-clockwise rotation of the transducer, which will make a right arch appear to descend on the left. The direction of the ascending aorta is not a reliable indicator of the side of the aortic arch. This is illustrated by a patient with dextrocardia whose arch passes to the left initially but descends to the right of the trachea with mirror-image branching (Figure 6–3).

ANOMALOUS SUBCLAVIAN ARTERY

With a left or right aortic arch the contralateral subclavian artery may arise anomalously as the last aortic arch branch rather than with the innominate artery

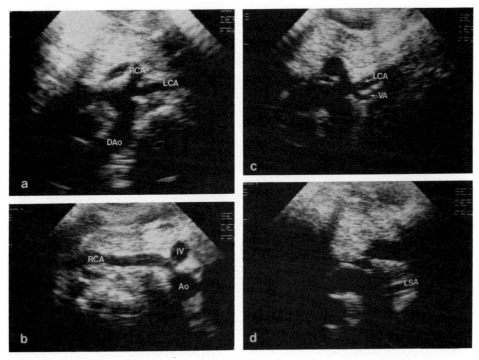

FIG. 6–5. Ultrasound imaging of abnormal branching of a left aortic arch. The patient has an anomalous right subclavian artery, as evidenced by the lack of normal right innominate artery (a), and in addition has the minor anomaly of origin of the left carotid artery (LCA) from the right carotid (RCA). A small left vertebral artery (VA) can be seen arising from the left carotid artery (c). The left subclavian artery originates in a normal location (d).

as the first branch. This results in a subclavian artery that passes from the descending aorta on the side of the arch to the opposite side *behind* the esophagus and trachea. The first clue to this anomaly during aortic arch scanning is the absence of normal branching of the first aortic arch branch. Scans posterior to this location image the subclavian artery passing toward the arm (Figure 6–4). The retroesophageal course of this vessel can be confirmed by imaging of the esophagus during swallowing.

An example of abnormal arch branching with a right aortic arch and anomalous origin of the left subclavian artery is shown in Figure 6–5. Here the origin of the left carotid artery from the right carotid artery, another abnormality, must be distinguished from normal branching of a right innominate artery. The vertebral artery arises abnormally but should not be confused with one of the major brachiocephalic arteries because of its smaller size.

VASCULAR RING

A wide variety of vascular rings can occur, but the two groups of greatest clinical significance as a cause of stridor in the infant are those involving the aortic arch and the fourth and sixth aortic arch derivatives[1] and the pulmonary

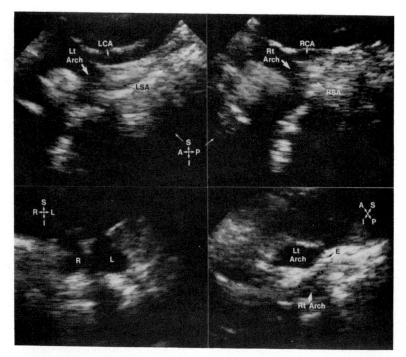

FIG. 6–6. Ultrasound imaging of double aortic arch. Note the similarities of the right-sided (upper left panel) and left-sided (upper right panel) aortic arch scans, scanning from the right to the left from the suprasternal position. A coronal scan (lower left panel) shows the common origin of these arches from the ascending aorta. The retroesophageal location of the right aortic arch is confirmed during esophageal visualization (lower right panel).

artery sling. In the former, persistence of some segments and regression of others lead to the most common vascular rings: double aortic arch and right aortic arch with anomalous left subclavian artery and a ligamentum. In a recent prospective study of 22 infants with stridor examined by ultrasonography, vascular ring as a cause of stridor was detected correctly in all eight shown to have it and was excluded in the others.

Double aortic arch can be diagnosed by cross-sectional imaging techniques[5] and is surgically remediable. From a suprasternal approach, the right-sided arch and its accompanying right carotid and subclavian arteries are imaged to the right of the esophagus. The left-sided arch appears similar to the right at the left of the esophagus (Figure 6–6). The course of the retroesophageal arch can be appreciated during esophageal visualization with swallowing of liquid.

The other common type of vascular ring is illustrated in Figure 6–7. A right aortic arch with anomalous left subclavian artery and Kommerell's diverticulum form a ring when there is a patent ductus arteriosus or ligamentum. Doppler techniques are useful in making this diagnosis.

OBSTRUCTION

Arch obstruction is unusual in the child and the most common congenital cause is interrupted aortic arch. Three principal types of aortic arch interruption

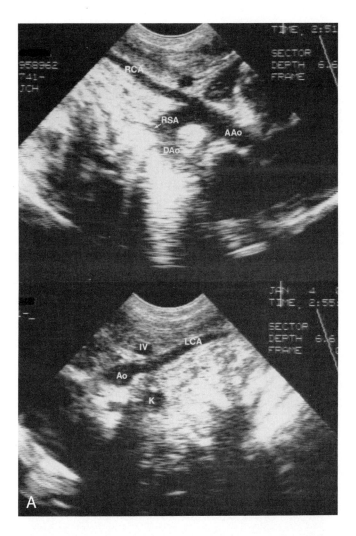

FIG. 6–7. Ultrasound imaging of a vascular ring formed by a right aortic arch with anomalous subclavian artery from a Kommerell's diverticulum with a patent ductus arteriosus. Scanning toward the right shoulder, (A) the aortic arch is seen to arise in a mirror image fashion with the descending aorta on the right, and the left carotid artery arises as a solitary vessel, suggesting anomalous origin of the left subclavian artery (B). The Kommerell's diverticulum (K) is seen coursing in a retroesophageal location (C). The vascular ring is completed by the patent ductus arteriosus, which was detected by Doppler ultrasonography (bottom).

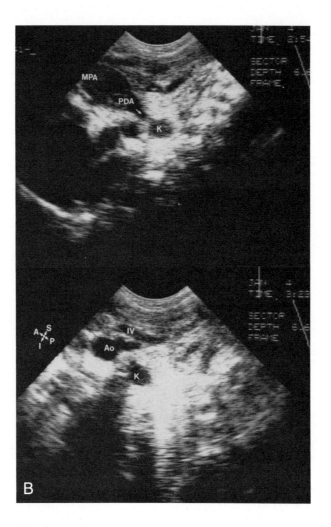

FIG. 6–7B *Continued.*

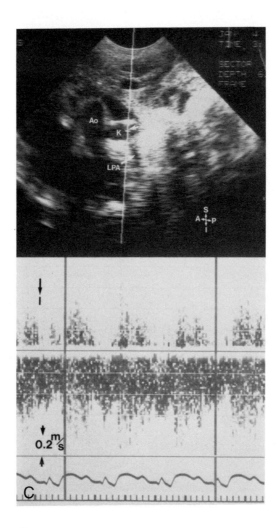

FIG. 6–7C *Continued.*

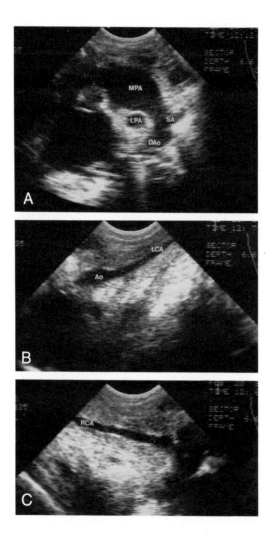

FIG. 6–8. Ultrasound imaging of interrupted aortic arch between the left carotid and left subclavian arteries, with anomalous origin of the right subclavian artery. Each of the respective carotid arteries arises as a solitary vessel (B and C), and there is a large ductus arteriosus connecting the main pulmonary artery and the descending aorta (A).

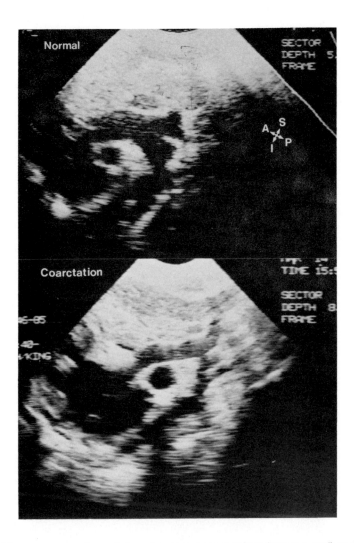

FIG. 6–9. Transverse aortic arch imaging in a normal infant (upper panel) and an infant with coarctation (lower panel). (From Morrow WR, Huhta JC, Murphy DJ, and McNamara DG: Quantitative morphology of the aortic arch in neonatal coarctation. J Am Coll Cardiol [in press]).

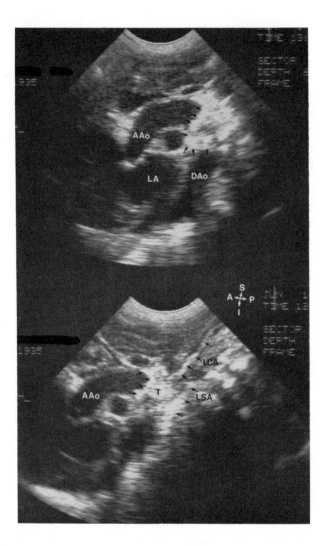

FIG. 6–10.   Ultrasound imaging of aortic arch thrombosis in a neonate. Note the extension of thrombogenic material, which is echodense, into the carotid and subclavian arteries.

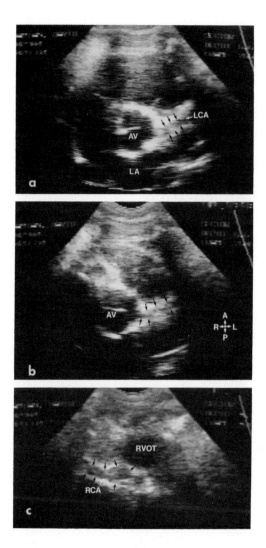

FIG. 6–11. A–C: Imaging of the proximal coronary arteries in a patient with Kawasaki's disease showing dilation typical of coronary artery aneurysms. (From Vargo TA, Huhta JC, Moore WH, et al: Recurrent Kawasaki syndrome. Pediatr Cardiol [in press]).

are based on location: distal to the innominate artery (type C), distal to the left carotid artery (type B), and distal to the left subclavian artery (type A).[1] The most common of these is interruption between the left carotid and left subclavian arteries (Figure 6–8) and is highly associated with DiGeorge's syndrome and abnormalities of the thymus (see Chapter 13). Early reports of ultrasound imaging of interrupted arch type B show the feasibility of noninvasive diagnosis in this condition.[6,7] In these very ill neonates the ductus arteriosus supplies the descending aorta (see Chapter 8), and there is usually a large ventricular septal defect. The ascending aorta is often hypoplastic (see Chapter 5) and has a vertical orientation. In terms of surgical treatment, it is important for the examiner to image the details of the arch branching and the distance that must be bridged in the repair.

The transverse aortic arch may be hypoplastic, with coarctation of the aorta (Chapter 7). The appearance of this area may aid in this diagnosis (Figure 6–9), due to the dramatic reduction in size compared to the ascending aorta.

ACQUIRED ABNORMALITIES

Obstruction of the aortic arch by thrombosis may be acquired either late in gestation or shortly after birth, and this rare condition resembles neonatal coarctation of the aorta.[8] Suprasternal imaging reveals normal aortic arch morphology, with obstruction of the arch by highly ultrasound-reflective material (Figure 6–10).

Aneurysmal dilation of the aortic arch or its branches is associated with mucocutaneous lymph node syndrome (Kawasaki's disease). Multiple, discrete aneurysms of the coronary and other arteries, including the brachiocephalic vessels, can occur and result in obstruction or stenosis as late sequelae. Careful examination of the coronary arteries is possible in children using cross-sectional ultrasound techniques for the detection of coronary artery aneurysms (Figure 6–11). In addition, the aortic arch arteries should be checked on each examination of these patients.

REFERENCES

1. Stewart JR, Kincaid OW, and Edwards JE: An Atlas of Vascular Rings and Related Malformations of the Aortic Arch System. Springfield, Ill: Charles C Thomas, 1964.
2. Tajik AJ, Seward JB, Hagler DJ, et al: Two-dimensional real-time ultrasonic imaging of the heart and great vessels: Technique, image orientation, structure identification, and validation. Mayo Clin Proc 53:271, 1978.
3. Huhta JC, Gutgesell HP, Latson LA, and Huffines FD: Two-dimensional echocardiographic assessment of the aorta in infants and children with congenital heart disease. Circulation 70:417, 1984.
4. Snider AR, and Silverman NH: Suprasternal notch echocardiography: A two-dimensional technique for evaluating congenital heart disease. Circulation 63:165, 1981.
5. Sahn DJ, Valdes-Cruz LM, Ovitt TW, et al: Two dimensional echocardiography and intravenous digital video substraction angiography for diagnosis and evaluation of double aortic arch. Am J Cardiol 50:342, 1982.
6. Riggs TW, Berry TE, Aziz KU, and Paul MH: Two-dimensional echocardiographic features of interruption of the aortic arch. Am J Cardiol 50:1385, 1982.

7. Smallhorn JF, Anderson RH, and Macartney FJ: Cross-sectional echocardiographic recognition of interruption of aortic arch between left carotid and subclavian arteries. Br Heart J 48:229, 1982.
8. Corrigan JJ Jr, Jeter M, Allen HD, and Malone JM: Aortic thrombosis in a neonate: Failure of urokinase thrombolytic therapy. Am J Pediatr Hematol Oncol 4:243, 1982.

chapter **7**

AORTIC ISTHMUS AND DESCENDING AORTA

The isthmus portion of the aorta is the most difficult to examine by means of cross-sectional ultrasound. This is true because it is in a transition portion of the aorta, between the arch, which passes leftward and posterior, and the descending aorta, which passes inferior. Scans of the ascending aorta or the aortic arch fail to properly examine the isthmus because of their very different planes.[1] The normal aortic isthmus is in a nearly sagittal plane, and scanning of this region should not include any arch structures except the left subclavian artery (Plate XV, and Figure 7–1). Both suprasternal and high parasternal sagittal scans allow visualization of this region (Figure 7–2). By investigating the tomographic anatomy of the isthmus, the pioneering work of Smallhorn and Anderson[2] paved the way for routine imaging of this area in the neonate. Careful attention to positioning the neonate with a small roll behind the shoulders results in slight extension of the neck so that the suprasternal approach can be utilized. In the older child, a transducer position immediately below the left clavicle with the patient sitting up will usually give good results (see Chapter 1).

THE NORMAL AORTIC ISTHMUS

There is variability in the morphology of the normal isthmus, depending on the age of the patient. Shortly after birth, this region may superficially appear

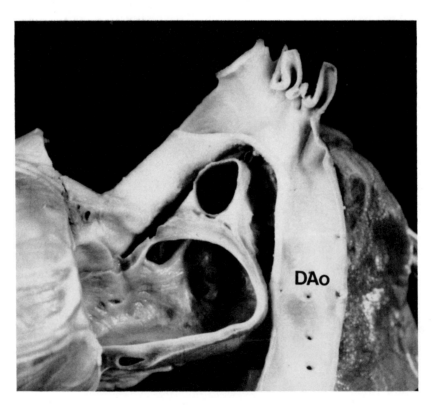

FIG. 7–1. Pathologic specimen of aortic isthmus and descending aorta (DAo) corresponding to Plate XV.

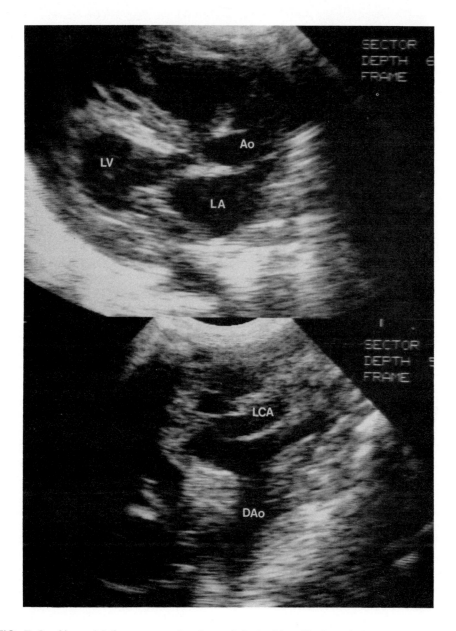

FIG. 7–2. Normal isthmus scanning in an infant with critical aortic stenosis excluding coarctation.

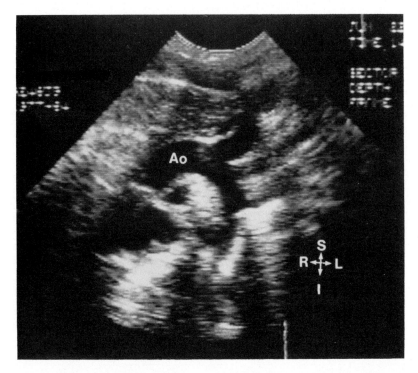

FIG. 7–3. Ultrasound imaging of the normal aortic isthmus. An anterior indentation may result from the entry site of the ductus arteriosus, and echodensity in the isthmus on scans including the ascending aorta are not related to the presence or absence of coarctation of the aorta.

narrowed (Figure 7–3), presumably because of low isthmus blood flow in utero. Actual observations of the isthmus in the human fetus suggest that this channel may be more important for flow than has been suggested by research in fetal lambs.[3] However, measurements of flow velocity in the newborn by a "pullback" across the isthmus by Doppler techniques show systolic turbulence. This mild narrowing is abolished by subsequent development of the isthmus with age and gradual obliteration of the region of the ductus arteriosus (see Chapter 8).

Little information is available concerning the normal diameter of the aortic isthmus at various ages. In the newborn infant the differential diagnosis of normal versus mild coarctation of the aorta is aided by this measurement (see below). Ultrasound measurements of the isthmus in the newborn in our laboratory range from 3.5 mm to 6.5 mm (mean = 4.1 mm + 0.8 mm).

It has been shown that the region of the aortic isthmus may contain ductus arteriosus tissue, which may contract after birth.[5] We have not observed such changes in normal newborns.

COARCTATION

Coarctation of the aorta is the most common abnormality affecting the aortic isthmus and has a wide morphologic spectrum. Classically these differences

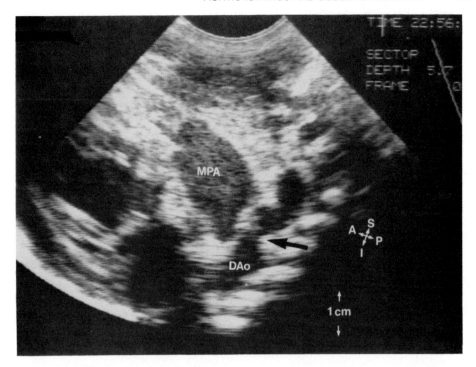

FIG. 7–4. Ultrasound imaging of coarctation of the aorta in a 2.7 kg infant. Note the posterior ledge impinging on the isthmus, (black arrow) which produces coarctation of the aorta.

have been divided into preductal, juxtaductal, and postductal coarctation. Most authors agree that the sine qua non of coarctation of the aorta is the posterior ledge.[6] This is a thin fibrous membrane protruding from the posterior aspect of the aorta; it is most often oriented toward the ductus arteriosus (juxtaductal coarctation) and obstructs flow from the upper to lower portions of the descending aorta. However, often left-to-right shunting occurs via a patent ductus arteriosus from the preductal area to the main pulmonary artery. This can be seen during aortography in neonatal coarctation and can be confirmed by Doppler sampling at the pulmonary end of the ductus (see Chapter 8).

The site of the ledge in relation to the ductus arteriosus forms the basis for many morphologic descriptions. It is possible to differentiate these various types by cross-sectional ultrasound imaging,[7] and these techniques are now being applied widely (Figure 7–4). A typical finding of neonatal coarctation of the aorta is narrowing and elongation of the transverse aorta between the left carotid and left subclavian arteries (Figure 7–5). It is thought that this is merely a reflection of decreased aortic isthmus flow in utero and is similar to the decreased diameter and increased length of any developing structure that experiences decreased flow. In normal neonates this distance ranges from 1.0 to 8.5 mm (mean 3.9), and in isolated neonatal coarctation the range is 6.0 to 12.5 mm (mean 8.8), $p < 0.0001$.

In older children with coarctation of the aorta there usually is marked medial deviation of the aortic isthmus, causing potential difficulty in imaging this region in one tomographic plane. In this situation it is necessary to scan the isthmus

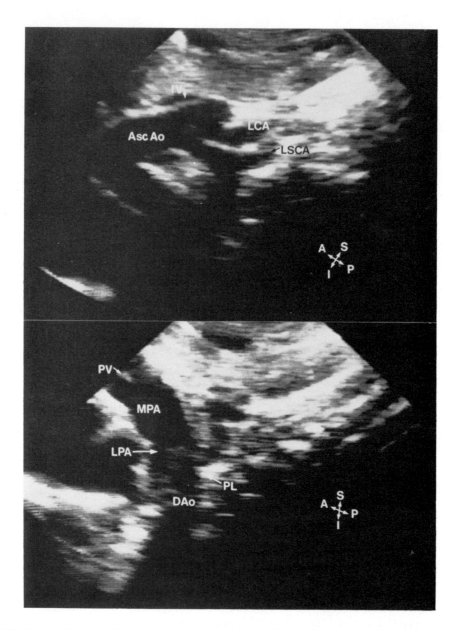

FIG. 7–5.   Ultrasound imaging of neonatal coarctation illustrating the associated elongation of the transverse aortic arch between the left carotid (LCA) and left subclavian arteries (LSA) (upper panel). The posterior ledge (PL) is also imaged from the isthmal scan (lower panel). (PV) = pulmonary valve.

and upper descending aorta from suprasternal and high sagittal approaches. A helpful finding in all such patients is the marked discrepancy between the pulsatility of the ascending aorta and the arch branches and the absence of pulsation below the isthmus and in the abdominal aorta. This lack of abdominal aortic pulsation is a useful observation in the fussy child, in whom accurate blood pressure measurements are difficult. This decrease in aortic pulsatility can be documented by M-mode echocardiographic imaging of the aorta just below the diaphragm.

There is a spectrum of possible origins of the left subclavian artery in coarctation. The subclavian artery may arise above, at, or below the level of the ductus arteriosus and posterior ledge. In cases of "atypical" coarctation, the left subclavian artery may arise distal to the posterior ledge (Figure 7–6), requiring some slight alteration in the technique of surgical repair. In a recent review of cross-sectional imaging of coarctation at the center, this type of anatomy was correctly diagnosed preoperatively in two children, and both had surgery without prior cardiac catheterization with a good result.

Doppler ultrasound in isolated coarctation in the neonate and infant is useful to (1) confirm the presence of obstruction by the posterior ledge, (2) diagnose patency of the ductus arteriosus, and (3) exclude coexisting aortic valve stenosis and assess the cardiac output.

TUBULAR HYPOPLASIA

The narrowing of the transverse arch or isthmus associated with coarctation may be quite severe and is often called *tubular hypoplasia*. This term has been applied to any decrease in size of either the arch or isthmus with coarctation but should be reserved for the rare case of severe, surgically significant hypoplasia (Figure 7–7). This type of hypoplasia has been described as affecting either portion of the transverse arch, the isthmus, or, rarely, is the substrate for "coarctation" without a well-developed posterior ledge (Figure 7–8). In neonates with isolated coarctation of the aorta, the transverse arch ranges from 2.5 to 4.5 mm (mean 3.5), while in normals the range is 4.5 to 6.5 mm (mean 5.5), $p < 0.0001$. Clinically, there is rarely a cuff blood pressure gradient between the arms, and this area of "hypoplasia" enlarges appropriately following adequate relief of the aortic obstruction.

In neonates with hypoplasia of the aortic isthmus, there frequently is coexisting pulmonary hypertension. There appears to be an inverse correlation between the size of the aortic isthmus and the degree of pulmonary hypertension from coarctation.

COARCTATION WITH VENTRICULAR SEPTAL DEFECT

When coarctation of the aorta is associated with a defect of the ventricular septum, nearly all such neonates present in the first month after birth with severe congestive heart failure and failure to thrive.[8] In general, the coarctation of the aorta and the hypoplasia of the aortic arch are more severe in this entity compared with isolated coarctation. When the defect is large and extends into

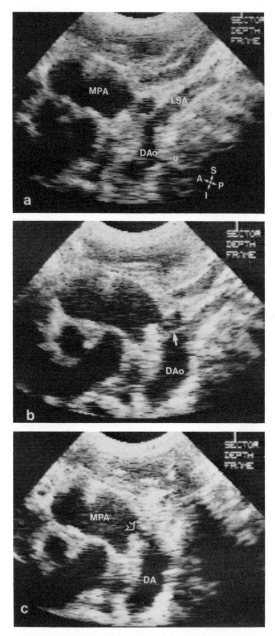

FIG. 7–6. Imaging of atypical coarctation with origin of the left subclavian artery distal to the coarctation ledge (a) and (b). The patent ductus (open white arrow) is seen in scanning more anteriorly (c). (From Glasow PF, Huhta JC, Murphy DJ Jr, et al: Surgery without angiography in abnormalities of the aorta in infancy. [Submitted for publication]).

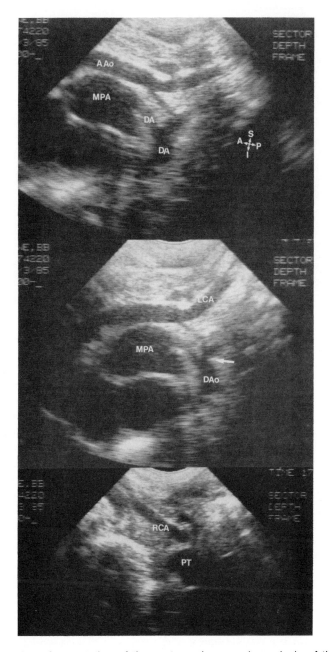

FIG. 7–7. Imaging of coarctation of the aorta and severe hypoplasia of the transverse aortic arch (upper panel). There is a posterior ledge of coarctation (white arrow, middle panel). There was anomalous origin of the right subclavian artery (lower panel). The surgical treatment required was similar to that for interrupted aortic arch. (From Glasow PF, Huhta JC, Murphy DJ Jr, et al: Surgery without angiography in abnormalities of the aorta in infancy. [Submitted for publication]).

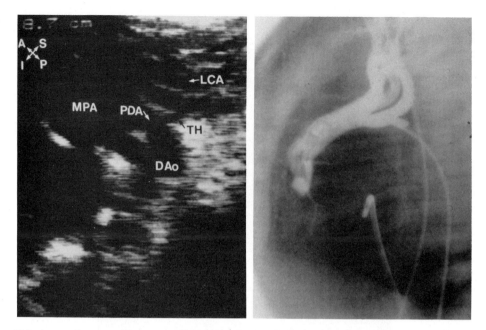

FIG. 7–8.   Severe tubular hypoplasia (TH) of the isthmus with a large patent ductus arteriosus in an infant with tricuspid atresia. Compare echocardiographic (left) and angiographic findings (right).

the outlet portion of the ventricular septum, there may be deviation of the subaortic infundibular septum muscle, causing the anatomic substrate for subaortic stenosis. This is similar to the ventricular septal anatomy found in interrupted aortic arch and has been implicated as a possible etiologic factor in the coarctation. The decreased ratio of the transverse aorta to the main pulmonary artery and the difference in distance between the left carotid and the left subclavian artery are exaggerated in this lesion (Figure 7–9). When there is doubt about the hemodynamic significance of the coarctation, Doppler (continuous wave or pulsed) examination from the suprasternal region may be useful to detect a patent ductus and a continuous, inferiorly directed jet with diastolic runoff (Figure 7–10).

COMPLEX COARCTATION

Coarctation of the aorta may be associated with complex congenital heart disease of several types. Neonates with tricuspid atresia and transposition of the great arteries or with double-inlet ventricle and the aorta arising from an outlet chamber with subaortic obstruction often have associated coarctation. In the evaluation of these patients it is mandatory that any subaortic obstruction be detected prior to any attempt at palliative surgery (Figure 7–11). Doppler sampling is useful to exclude any significant ventricle to aorta gradient and to estimate the Qp/Qs (Figure 7–12).

At the end of this spectrum of left-sided heart obstructive lesions is hypoplastic left-sided heart syndrome. In this condition there is frequently a hypoplastic

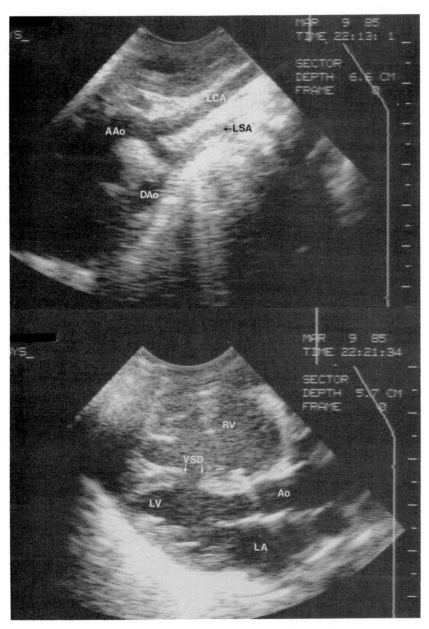

FIG. 7–9. Ultrasound imaging of coarctation of the aorta associated with a ventricular septal defect (VSD). The posterior ledge of coarctation cannot be seen clearly, but there is transverse aortic arch hypoplasia. A large ventricular septal defect is usually associated with this combination (lower panel).

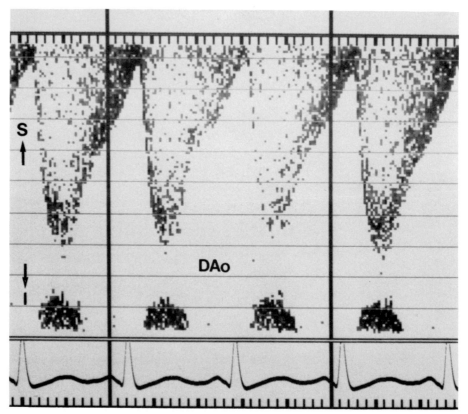

FIG. 7–10. Doppler sampling above the aortic isthmus in coarctation showing diastolic continuous flow velocity inferiorly.

isthmus, and some neonates have coarctation with a bona fide posterior ledge. The flow in the isthmal region is from the ductus retrograde around the arch, as there is aortic atresia and reversed flow only in the isthmus (Figure 7–13). In such lesions the aortic isthmus appears to insert in the ductus, which is supplying the descending aorta. Pathologic reports of series of patients with hypoplastic left-sided heart syndrome are conflicting regarding the incidence of coarctation. It is likely that, with ductus closure, this area becomes severely stenotic even without a posterior ledge.

DESCENDING AORTA

The thoracic and abdominal portions of the descending aorta can be evaluated with ultrasonography using parasternal and subcostal scans (Plate XVI).

Visualization of the entire retrocardiac course may require moving the patient to the left lateral position and scanning segmentally, taking one portion at a time (Figure 7–14). The abdominal descending aorta is well visualized using subcostal scans (see Figure 2–13).

Abnormalities of the descending aorta are uncommon in pediatrics. Diagnosis

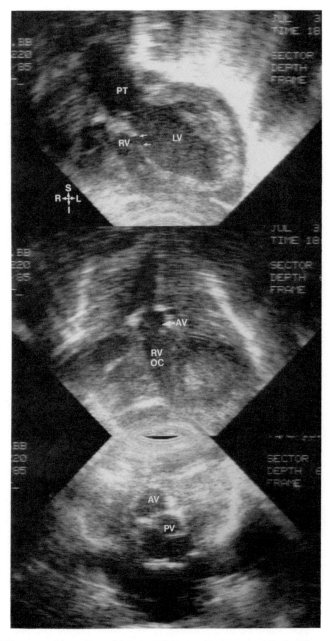

FIG. 7–11. Ultrasound imaging of intracardiac anatomy associated with complex coarctation of the aorta with double inlet ventricle and subaortic stenosis (white arrows). The aortic valve (AV) was anterior and to the right of the pulmonary trunk (lower panel). RVOC = right ventricular subaortic outlet chamber. (From Glasow PF, Huhta JC, Murphy DJ Jr, et al: Surgery without angiography in abnormalities of the aorta in infancy. [Submitted for publication]).

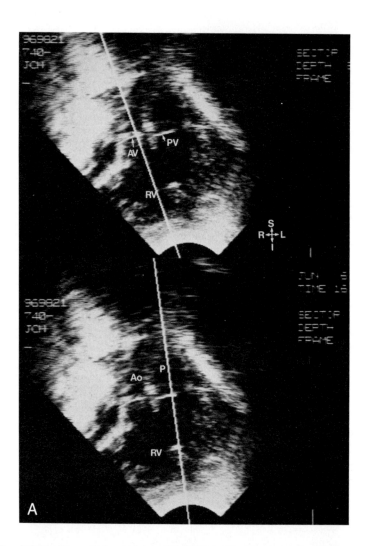

FIG. 7–12. (A) Double-outlet ventricle with side-by-side great arteries illustrating the technique of aortic (upper panel) and pulmonary (lower panel) pulsed Doppler sampling from the subcostal position. (B) Doppler tracings show no evidence of subaortic stenosis and the pulmonary velocity integral is greater than the aortic, suggestive of a large Qp/Qs.

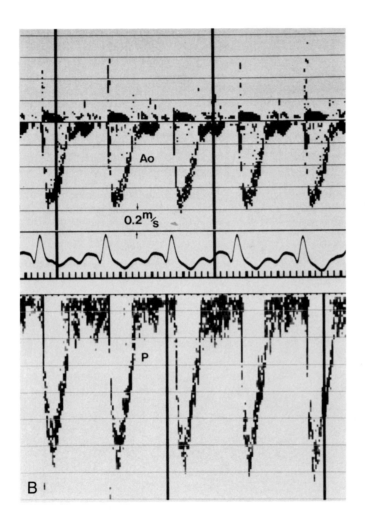

FIG. 7–12 *Continued.*

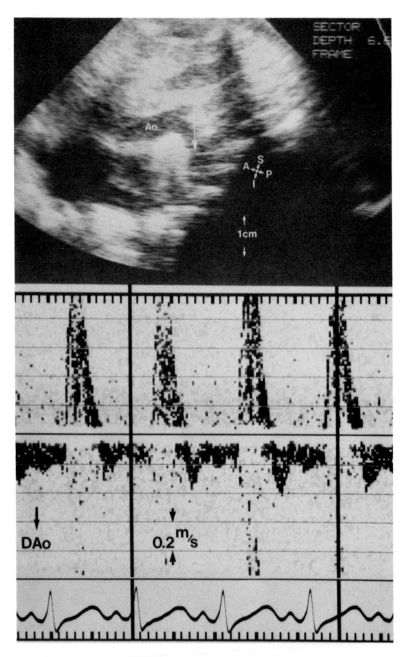

FIG. 7–13. Pulsed Doppler sampling at the site of the arrow in hypoplastic left heart syndrome with aortic atresia, showing reversed systolic isthmal flow.

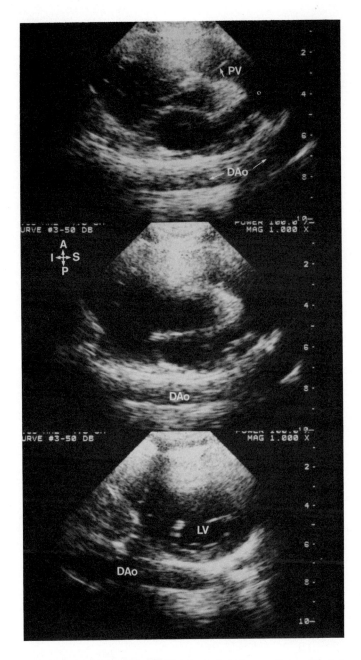

FIG. 7–14. Sagittal scans of the descending aorta (upper panel) near the isthmus, (middle panel) at its midthoracic level, and (lower panel) near the diaphragm.

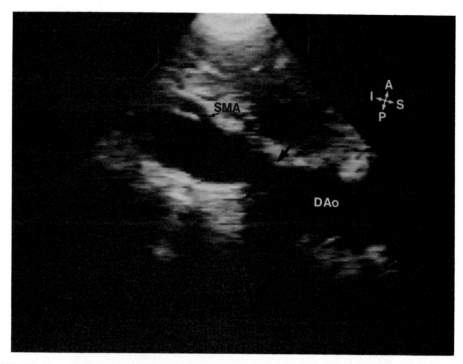

FIG. 7–15. Abdominal aortic obstruction (black arrow) in a child with Takayasu's disease.

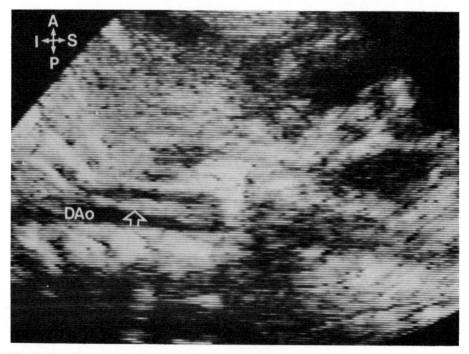

FIG. 7–16. Subcostal sagittal scan of the descending aorta (DAo), which contains a thrombus related to an umbilical artery catheter (open white arrow).

of abdominal coarctation by ultrasonography has been reported,[10,11] and acquired descending aorta obstruction may be diagnosed noninvasively (Figure 7–15). When an umbilical artery catheter is used in a newborn baby, there is always a risk of residual thrombosis after the catheter is removed (Figure 7–16).[12]

REFERENCES

1. Huhta JC, Gutgesell HP, Latson LA, and Huffines FD: Two-dimensional echocardiographic assessment of the aorta in infants and children with congenital heart disease. Circulation 70:417, 1984.
2. Smallhorn JF, Huhta JC, Anderson RH, and Macartney FJ: Suprasternal cross-sectional echocardiography in the assessment of patent ductus arteriosus. Br Heart J 48:321, 1982.
3. Huhta JC, Vick GW, Carpenter RA, and Gutgesell HP: Transient neonatal tricuspid regurgitation: Possible relation with premature closure of the ductus arteriosus. (Letter to the Editor.) J Am Coll Cardiol 4:651, 1984.
4. Ho SY, and Anderson RH: Coarctation, tubular hypoplasia, and the ductus arteriosus. Histological study of 35 specimens. Br Heart J 41:268, 1979.
5. Huhta JC, Cohen M, and Gutgesell HP: Patency of the ductus arteriosus in normal neonates: Two-dimensional echocardiography versus Doppler assessment. J Am Coll Cardiol 4:561, 1984.
6. Duncan WJ, Ninomiya K, Cook DH, and Rowe RD: Noninvasive diagnosis of neonatal coarctation and associated anomalies using two-dimensional echocardiography. Am Heart J 106:63, 1983.
7. Smallhorn JF, Huhta JC, Adams PS, et al: Cross-sectional echocardiographic assessment of coarctation in the sick neonate and infant. Br Heart J 50:349, 1983.
8. Smallhorn JF, Anderson RH, and Macartney FJ: Morphological characterization of ventricular septal defects associated with coarctation of aorta by cross-sectional echocardiography. Br Heart J 49:485, 1983.
9. Come PC: Improved cross-sectional echocardiographic technique for visualization of the retrocardiac descending aorta in its long axis. Am J Cardiol 51:1029, 1983.
10. Saveuse N, Goupil-Colliard M, Bacourt F, and Tcherdakoff P: [Coarctation of the abdominal aorta: Diagnosis, pathogenesis, medical or surgical treatment. 7 cases]. Presse-Med 12:1475, 1983.
11. Scott HW Jr, Dean RH, Boerth R, et al: Coarctation of the abdominal aorta: Pathophysiologic and therapeutic considerations. Ann Surg 189:746, 1979.
12. George L, Waldman JD, Kirkpatrick SE, et al: Umbilical vascular catheters: localization by two-dimensional echocardio/aortography. Pediatr Cardiol 2:237, 1982.

chapter 8

DUCTUS ARTERIOSUS

The ductus arteriosus is a complex muscular structure connecting the main pulmonary artery and the descending aorta. In utero, the ductus arteriosus functions to shunt blood from the main pulmonary artery to the lower body, bypassing the pulmonary circulation where the pulmonary blood flow is low. Following birth, pulmonary blood flow increases and the ductus arteriosus closes spontaneously as a result of mechanisms that are not entirely clear but are related to the increase in arterial oxygen concentration and changes in the prostaglandin environment. The process of ductus closure involves initial constriction followed by structural change in the wall and lumen and eventually complete obliteration. The resulting structure is called the ligamentum arteriosum.

Isolated patency of the ductus arteriosus is a common form of congenital heart disease. Patency may be present in association with other congenital defects such as ventricular septal defect or pulmonary stenosis. Some forms of congenital heart disease are improved by a patent ductus arteriosus, such as neonatal coarctation of the aorta (see Chapter 7), pulmonary atresia, or hypoplastic left-sided heart syndrome. Manipulation of the ductus arteriosus pharmacologically using (1) prostaglandin derivatives in order to keep it open, or (2) prostaglandin inhibitors to close it has allowed further observation of *changes* in ductus structure by suprasternal ultrasonography.

IMAGING TECHNIQUE

The proper tomographic plane in which to image the normally oriented ductus arteriosus was delineated by Smallhorn and associates[1,2] (Plate XVII). With the infant or older child in the recumbent position and a pillow or roll under the shoulders, the head is allowed to fall back, giving access to the suprasternal notch. The transducer head is placed in the suprasternal notch or slightly to the right and superior of it. The plane of section needed in order to properly image the ductus arteriosus in its full length must transect the main and left pulmonary arteries and the descending aorta (Figure 8–1). In order for the examiner to hold this position for long periods of time, it is mandatory that he or she be seated (see Chapter 1).

DUCTUS ARTERIOSUS MORPHOLOGY

There is a broad spectrum of ductus arteriosus morphology, and this is de-termined in large part by the pattern of blood flow in utero prior to birth. As a result of recent advances in ultrasound imaging technology, the ductus arte-riosus can be imaged in the human fetus (Figure 8–2) and resembles a patent ductus in a premature infant.[3] The normal human ductus appears very similar before and after birth. The structure courses posteriorly, and slightly toward the left. Because blood flow is from the pulmonary artery into the descending aorta in utero, where it enters the upper descending aorta, the ductus forms an acute angle (Figure 8–3).

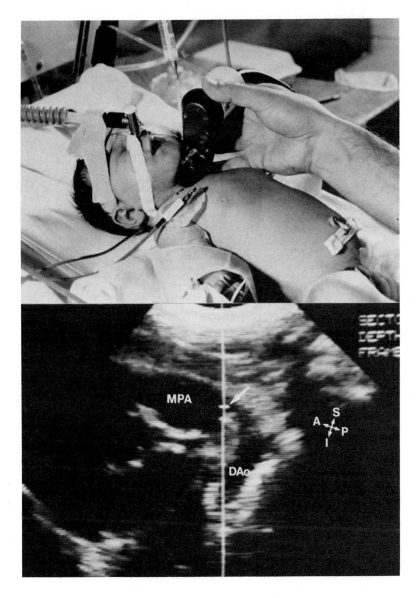

FIG. 8–1. Imaging of the ductus arteriosus from a suprasternal approach in an ill newborn infant. Pulsed Doppler sampling in the pulmonary end of the ductus arteriosus is illustrated in the lower panel (white arrow).

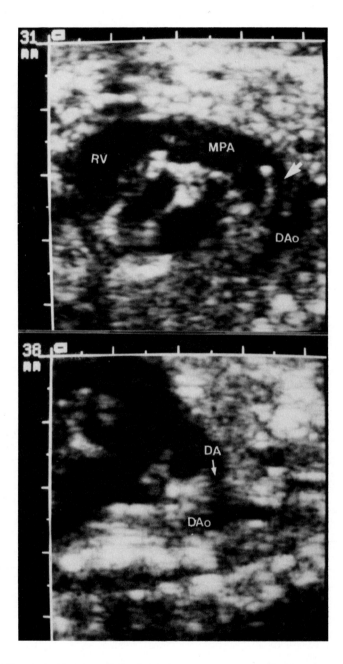

FIG. 8–2. Ultrasonic imaging of the fetal ductus arteriosus. (Reprinted with permission from the Journal of the American College of Cardiology. From Huhta JC, Vick GW, Carpenter RA, Gutgesell HP. Transient neonatal tricuspid regurgitation: Possible relation with premature closure of the ductus arteriosus. (Letter to the Editor.) J Am Coll Cardiol 4(3):651, 1984.)

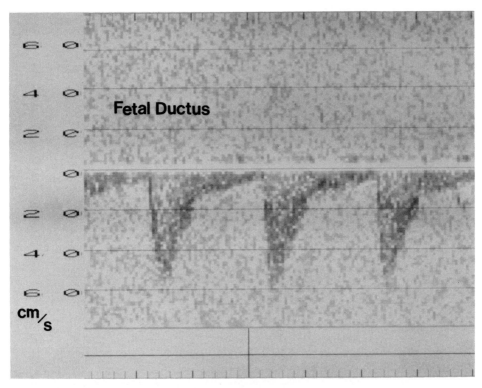

FIG. 8–3. Pulsed Doppler sampling in the fetal ductus arteriosus showing a systolic velocity with diastolic run-off in the same direction, toward the descending aorta. The peak velocity is approximately 60 cm/sec in this fetus of 20 weeks' gestation.

DUCTUS ARTERIOSUS IN THE NORMAL NEWBORN

Immediately after birth, the ductus arteriosus rapidly changes from a widely patent structure (Figure 8–4) to a narrowed, nearly closed aortic to pulmonary intercommunication. When directed by suprasternal two-dimensional (2-D) imaging of the ductus Doppler echocardiography is useful in assessing the hemodynamic effects. The flow pattern in the ductus arteriosus can be assessed from suprasternal or parasternal measurements in normal neonates. It is predominantly from the aorta to the pulmonary artery.[3,4] Soon after birth, when pulmonary pressure is high, the velocity peak of left-to-right shunting is attenuated. Within 24 hours, the combination of further ductus closure plus the normal drop in pulmonary artery pressure results in a pattern of higher frequency left-to-right shunting (Figure 8–5).[5] The closed ductus arteriosus manifests extensive obliteration of the ductus lumen.

DUCTUS ARTERIOSUS IN THE PREMATURE INFANT

In premature infants with lung disease, a patent ductus arteriosus may significantly alter the clinical course (Figure 8–6). The morphologic variability of

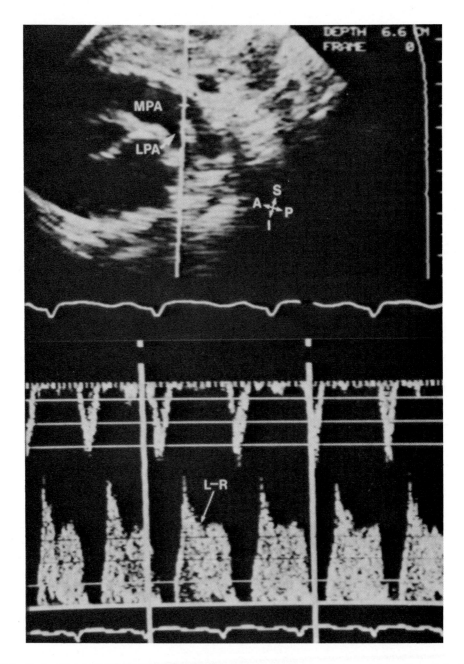

FIG. 8–4. Pulsed Doppler sampling in the ductus arteriosus of a normal newborn infant at two hours old. Note the bidirectional shunting with predominant left-to-right (L–R) shunt.

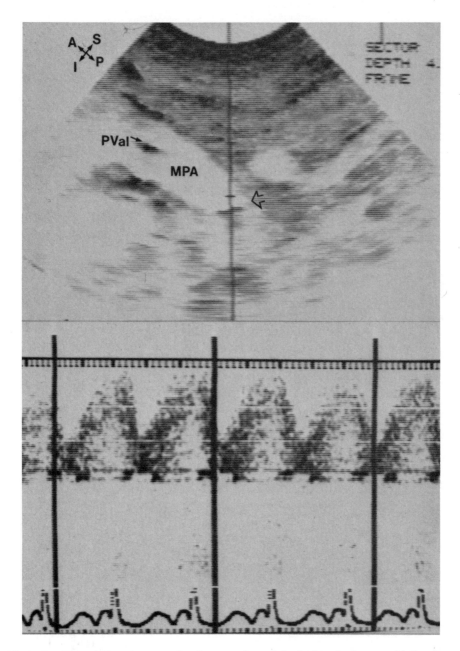

FIG. 8–5. Pulsed Doppler sampling in a newborn infant after ductus constriction (open white arrow) with a pattern of nearly continuous ductal shunting toward the transducer (PVal = pulmonary valve). (Reprinted with permission from the American College of Cardiology. J Am Coll Cardiol 4:561, 1984.)

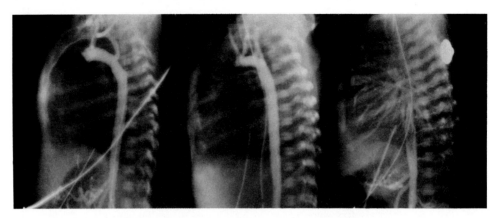

FIG. 8–6. Angiograms of the aorta of premature infants showing no PDA (left), a small shunt (middle), and a large shunt filling the pulmonary arteries (right).

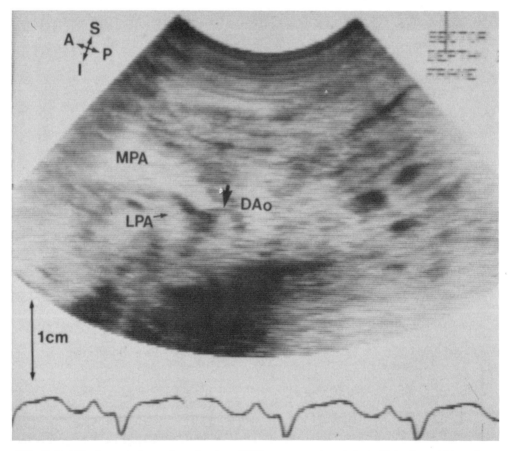

FIG. 8–7. Ductus arteriosus imaging in a 1000-gm premature infant. Note the midductal constriction (white arrow). There is patency of the pulmonary end of the ductus arteriosus but constriction of the midportion.

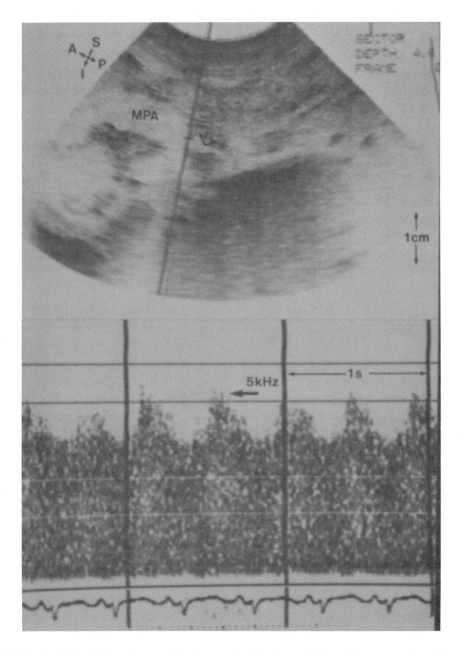

FIG. 8–8. Pulsed Doppler sampling in a patent ductus arteriosus in a premature infant. Note the continuous left-to-right shunting toward the transducer (lower panel).

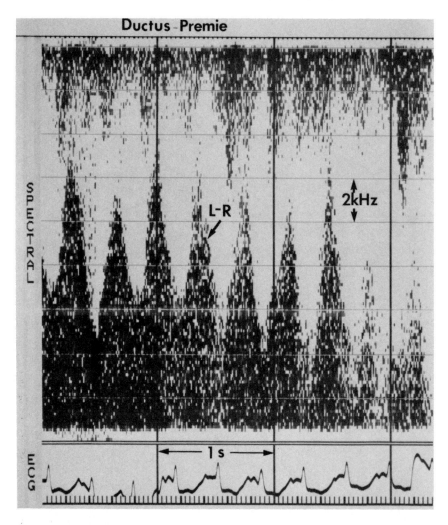

FIG. 8–9. Pulsed Doppler sampling in a premature ductus. Note the wide variation in peak velocity of the left-to-right shunt (L–R). It may be possible to estimate the pressure difference between the aorta and the pulmonary artery using this Doppler information.

the ductus arteriosus can be assessed by 7.5 MHz suprasternal echocardiography. It is possible by combined cross-sectional and Doppler techniques to differentiate the widely patent from the constricted patent ductus arteriosus (PDA). Imaging shows the midductal narrowing (Figure 8–7) and Doppler confirms continuous blood flow velocity (Figure 8–8).[8] It is hoped that these observations will correlate with responsiveness of the ductus arteriosus to closure by indomethacin, a pharmacologic constrictor. We speculate that this methodology will some day allow prediction of which premature infants should have early surgical ductus ligation when a widely patent ductus is present early in association with pulmonary disease (Figure 8–9).

In the premature infant it is not sufficient to use suprasternal echocardiography to prove that the ductus is patent. The magnitude of the left-to-right shunt is significant in relation to the effect of the ductus arteriosus on the lungs and on the systemic circulation. Qualitative severity of patent ductus effects can now be assessed noninvasively by mapping the radiation of diastolic runoff from the aorta into the pulmonary arteries. However, elevated pulmonary artery pressure caused by lung disease may modify these observations. Early data from studies at Texas Children's Hospital suggest that diastolic runoff into the proximal pulmonary arteries as assessed by suprasternal Doppler echocardiography indicates a significant left-to-right shunt. In addition, measurement of the pressure gradient across the ductus may be useful. Contrast echocardiography can be used to assess patency by injections in an umbilical artery catheter placed below the region of the ductus (Figure 8–10). Ultrasonic observations of ductus morphology after indomethacin treatment may be useful.

PDA IN OLDER CHILDREN AND ADULTS

It is not known what structural wall defect in the ductus arteriosus allows persistent patency, producing the classic patent ductus arteriosus. The resultant left-to-right shunt usually does not cause severe symptoms, and this defect often remains undetected in patients until later in childhood or adult life. There is some morphologic variability in PDA, with some patients having a widely patent aortic portion tapering to a stenotic pulmonary end and others manifesting discrete narrowing in the midportion between the aortic and pulmonary ends (Figure 8–11). There may be associated mitral insufficiency leading to further left atrial enlargement.

At Texas Children's Hospital, 20 patients have had prospective imaging of the ductus arteriosus followed by detailed angiography for the purpose of defining the internal structure of the ductus. The echocardiographic observations mentioned above were confirmed angiographically. The morphologic variability in the ductus arteriosus is of more than academic interest because these patients are possible candidates for transvenous closure. Because these patients all underwent an attempt at transvenous closure with an umbrella device, we used suprasternal echocardiography to predict the success of this procedure based on morphologic appearance. It was found that the procedure is more difficult to accomplish in the patient with a ductus arteriosus measuring 4 mm or more by echocardiography and that manifests little tapering from the pulmonary to the aortic end. The size of the narrowest portion of the PDA varied from 2 to 6 mm angiographically, and 2-D echocardiography was correlated with these findings and consistently underestimated this size. Therefore, suprasternal 2-D echocardiography may aid in the selection of patients for surgery rather than transvenous closure in the catheterization laboratory. This study also confirmed the observations of Smallhorn and associates[2] concerning the need to use the suprasternal approach to properly examine this structure. Doppler techniques are also useful in follow-up of patients with small residual shunts after ductal occlusion (Figures 8–12 and 8–13).

PDA WITH LARGE LEFT-TO-RIGHT SHUNT

A small PDA is common in association with ventricular septal defect or atrioventricular canal defect and can be difficult to diagnose by any technique except

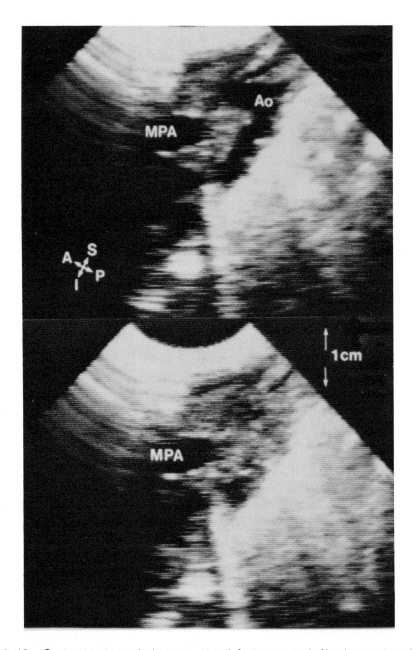

FIG. 8–10. Contrast aortography in a premature infant suspected of having a patent ductus arteriosus. Saline was injected into an umbilical artery catheter placed high in the thoracic aorta. Prior to injection (upper panel), there was no opacification of the aorta. After injection (lower panel), the aorta was completely opacified while the main pulmonary artery did not show echo-contrast, indicating a closed ductus arteriosus.

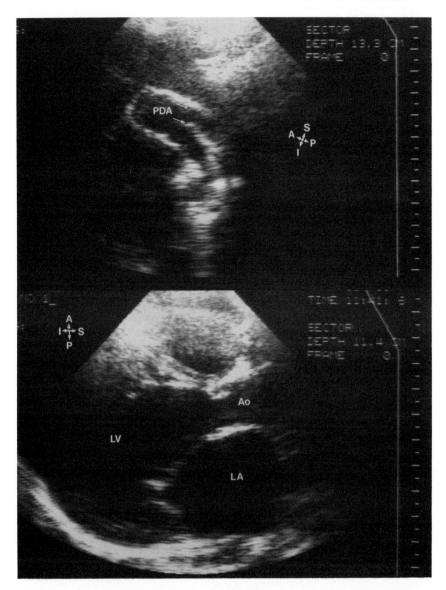

FIG. 8–11. Cross-sectional imaging of a large patent ductus arteriosus (upper panel). There was associated mitral valve disease with mitral insufficiency causing marked atrial enlargement on a parasternal scan of the left ventricle and left atrium (lower panel).

aortography. However, a large PDA in association with other congenital heart disease has considerable significance and should usually be ligated or divided prior to any attempt at complete surgical repair of other intracardiac defects. It is known that a large PDA may mimic a large ventricular septal defect or atrioventricular canal in an infant with severe congestive heart failure. We have had the experience in the last two years of treating six infants, aged two to three months, presenting with "viral pneumonia" and intractable congestive heart failure due to a patent ductus arteriosus. Two of these infants were chronically dependent on ventilator assistance. In each case, surgical ligation of the ductus

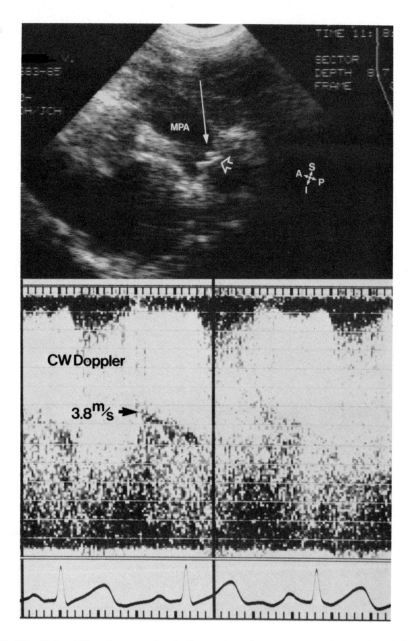

FIG. 8–12. Pulsed Doppler sampling in the main pulmonary artery in a patient following ductus arteriosus occlusion with an umbrella device (open arrow). There is persistent ductus patency with a peak diastolic velocity in the main pulmonary artery of 3.8 m/sec of the left-to-right shunt.

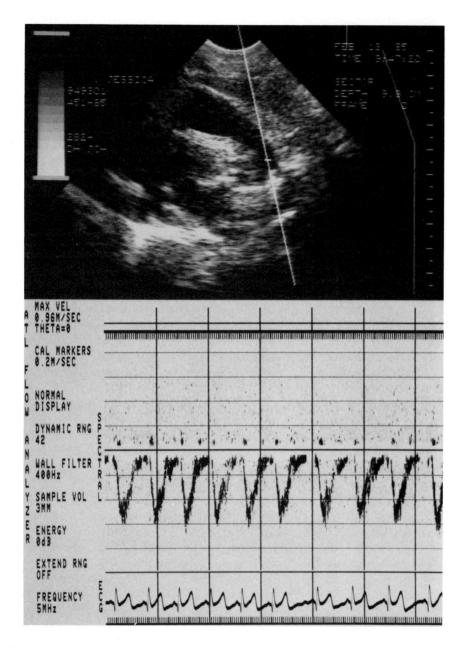

FIG. 8–13.   Pulsed Doppler sampling in the main pulmonary artery in a patient after ductus arteriosus umbrella occlusion showing no residual left-to-right shunt and a normal antegrade pulmonary blood flow velocity pattern.

arteriosus resulted in immediate improvement and discharge from the hospital in 10 days. The ability to confidently image the ductus arteriosus from suprasternal scans can be of great benefit in such infants, since it obviates the need for cardiac catheterization or angiography. Assessment of pulmonary artery pressure may be feasible by this technique (Figure 8–14). When there is pulmonary hypertension, M-mode and Doppler imaging may be useful (Figure 8–15).

In a consecutive series of 262 children with congenital heart disease, abnormalities of the aorta were predicted using cross-sectional imaging only. There were 57 children with a ductus arteriosus, and 53 were detected (sensitivity was 93%).[10] There were two false positive findings for ductus arteriosus.

DUCTUS ARTERIOSUS IN PULMONARY ATRESIA

In patients with decreased pulmonary blood flow attributable to severe pulmonary stenosis or pulmonary atresia, the ductus manifests a different morphology. In pulmonary valve atresia and ventricular septal defect, a left ductus from a left arch appears morphologically different (Figure 8–16A). Arising from under the transverse aortic arch, the ductus appears as a continuation of the aortic arch, curling back to supply the pulmonary arteries. In atresia of the pulmonary valve the ductal flow is presumably reversed in utero, so that ascending aortic blood flow courses from the aorta to the pulmonary arteries in the direction opposite that of normal. Imaging should confirm that confluent pulmonary arteries are supplied by the ductus (Figure 8–17).

In pulmonary atresia the ductus arteriosus usually is on the same side as the aortic arch, giving the pattern described above either on the left or right. A common situation with a right aortic arch is a left ductus arteriosus that originates from the left innominate artery and courses inferiorly to the junction of the main and left pulmonary arteries. Occasionally, bilateral ducti are present, and in this situation it is common to see coexisting nonconfluent right and left pulmonary arteries (Figure 8–18). A right ductus and a left arch can occur with bilateral ducti, as illustrated by a patient with "absent" right pulmonary artery (Figure 8–19). Bidirectional shunting was present, as seen by Doppler sampling in the left ductus (Figure 8–20). In order to completely diagnose this situation noninvasively, a systematic approach from the suprasternal notch is necessary to examine the aorta, aortic arch branches, pulmonary arteries, and ductus arteriosus.

In pulmonary atresia with intact ventricular septum, the ductus arteriosus morphology is variable but lies between the ductus arteriosus of pulmonary atresia with ventricular septal defect and that of normal. Originating from the descending aorta, as in normals, in this situation the ductus arteriosus has a more obtuse angle from the descending aorta when compared with the normal ductus, which has a relatively acute angle (Figure 8–16). In pulmonary atresia with intact ventricular septum, it is thought that pulmonary-to-aortic shunt via the ductus may occur in utero prior to the complete atresia of the valve orifice, resulting in this structural variability.

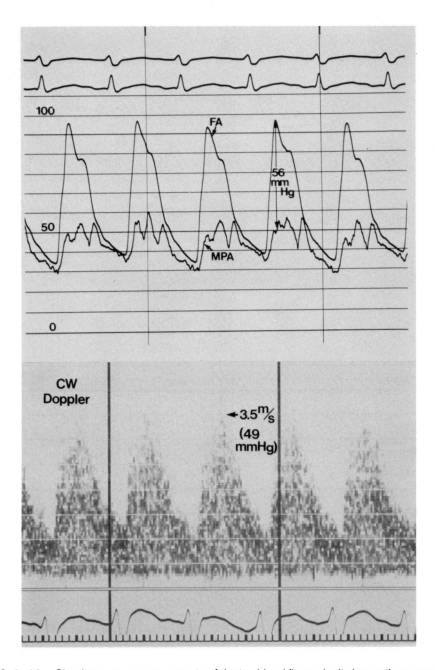

FIG. 8–14. Simultaneous measurements of ductus blood flow velocity by continuous wave Doppler (lower panel) and femoral artery and main pulmonary artery pressures. Note that the Doppler closely approximates the peak gradient across the ductus arteriosus.

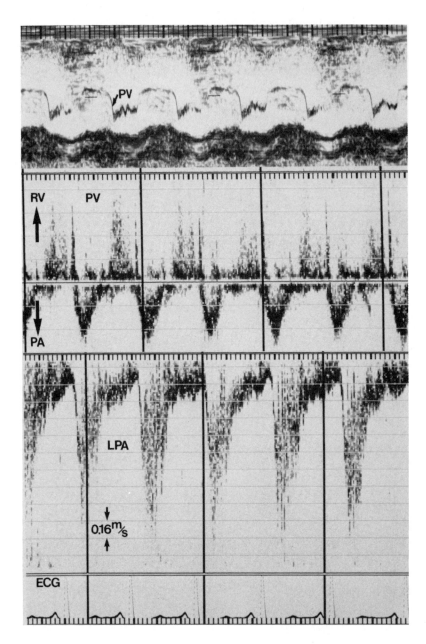

FIG. 8–15. M-mode echocardiography (upper panel) and pulsed Doppler (nonsimultaneous) at the pulmonary valve (middle panel) and left pulmonary artery (lower panel) in a child with a patent ductus arteriosus and severe pulmonary hypertension. Note the presence of pulmonary insufficiency sampling near the pulmonary valve.

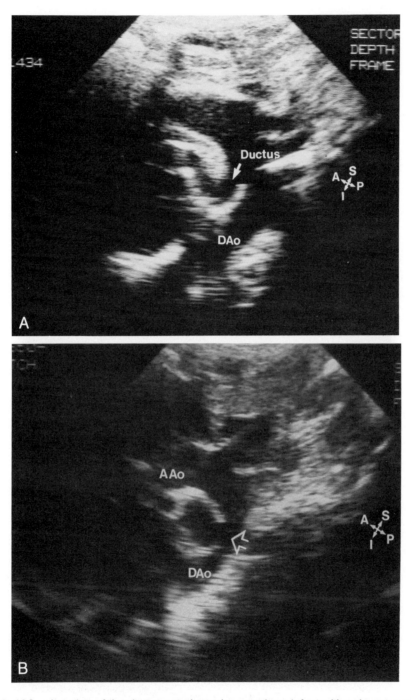

FIG. 8–16A.   Imaging of the ductus arteriosus in a newborn infant with pulmonary atresia and ventricular septal defect. Note the unusual morphology of the ductus, which originates from beneath the aortic arch; this is typical of pulmonary blood flow that was exclusively supplied by the ductus in utero. **B.** Ductus morphology in a neonate with pulmonary atresia and intact ventricular septum.

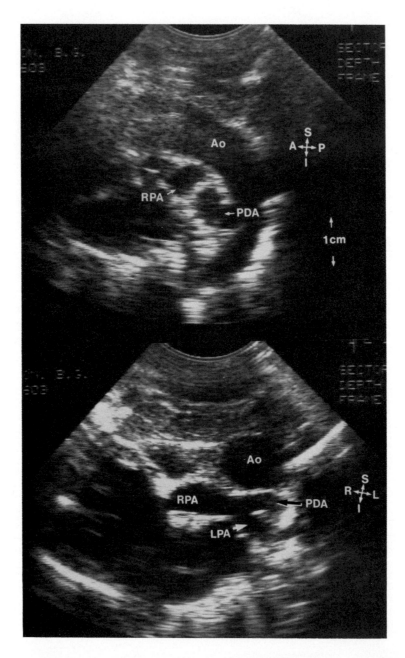

FIG. 8–17. Suprasternal imaging of a newborn infant with pulmonary atresia and a left ductus arteriosus (PDA). Confluent left and right pulmonary arteries are supplied by the ductus arteriosus (lower panel).

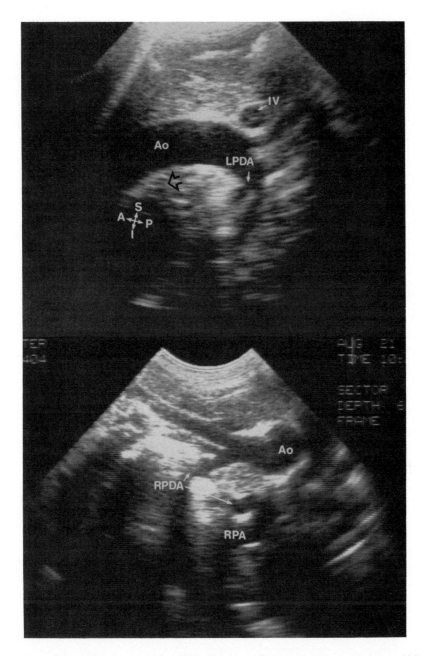

FIG. 8–18. Suprasternal scans of a child with nonconfluent pulmonary arteries and bilateral ductus arteriosus. The ascending aorta is normal, and a left patent ductus arteriosus (LPDA) is seen arising beneath the aortic arch. Note the absence of the normal right pulmonary artery or main pulmonary artery confluence (open black arrow), suggesting nonconfluent pulmonary arteries. Scanning toward the right shoulder (lower panel), a right patent ductus arteriosus (RPDA) is visualized, arising from the innominate artery.

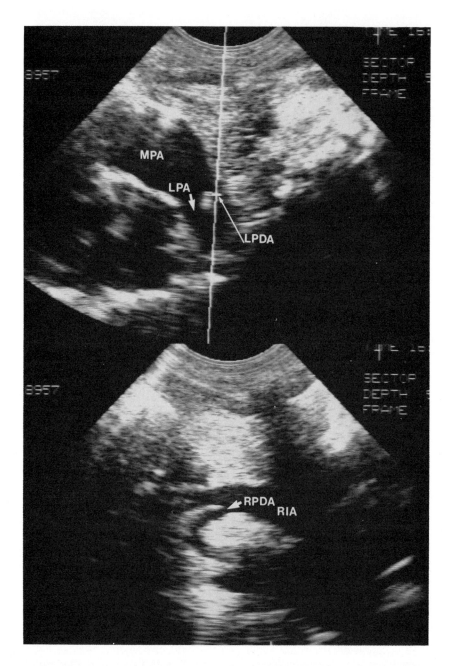

FIG. 8–19. Bilateral ducti in a patient with pulmonary hypertension and hypoplasia of the right lung. The right patent ductus arteriosus (RPDA) supplied only four segments of lung on the right.

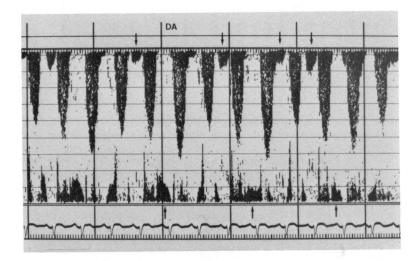

FIG. 8–20. Pulsed Doppler sampling in the patient illustrated in Figure 8–19 showing right-to-left ductus shunt through the left PDA. There was variability in the occurrence of bidirectional shunting relating to respiration (black arrows).

DUCTUS ARTERIOSUS IN TRANSPOSITION OF THE GREAT ARTERIES

With transposition of the great arteries, the aorta and pulmonary artery course parallel from the heart, and the ductus arteriosus comes to lie in a plane that is different from that of normals.[11] This greatly enhances the capability of complete ductus arteriosus examination from the suprasternal notch and high parasternal approaches (Figure 8–21). We have utilized the infant with transposition of the great arteries and intact ventricular septum as a model of ductus closure, observing the events combining ductus arteriosus constriction at the pulmonary end with later luminal obliteration. Early observations suggest that infolding of the ductus wall rather than thrombosis causes the observable echodensities to form. Figure 8–22 shows an example of a patient with a widely PDA on prostaglandin who had ductus closure following withdrawal of this medication. Twenty-four hours later it was necessary to readminister this medication because of severe cyanosis, and the ductus manifested residual narrowing. It appears that structural change in the ductus arteriosus may mediate prostaglandin responsiveness, and that changes in wall structure correlate with increased echodensity on suprasternal echocardiography. These densities appear intraluminal and correspond to the intimal "cushions" observed pathologically. Observations of ductus arteriosus opening and closing in this situation confirm the pathologic and clinical observations that the ductus normally constricts first in its midportion toward the pulmonary end.

It is useful to combine Doppler and 2-D imaging in assessment of the ductus arteriosus to detect patency. This may be done in the main pulmonary artery, preferably from the high parasternal approach or in the ductus (Figure 8–23).

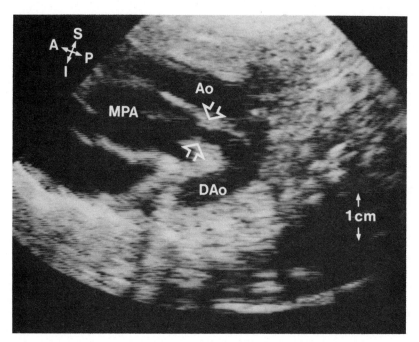

FIG. 8–21. Ductus arteriosus imaging from a suprasternal notch approach in a newborn infant with transposition of the great arteries. Note the ductus wall thickening related to constriction (open white arrows).

PDA IN COARCTATION OF THE AORTA

PDA with coarctation of the aorta or interrupted aortic arch may result in palliation of either lesion by shunting of blood from the main pulmonary artery to the lower body below the area of obstruction (see Chapter 7).[12] For this reason a widely patent ductus arteriosus may mask severe coarctation of the aorta or interrupted aortic arch by providing the lower body with near normal pulsatile flow.[7] Therefore, knowledge of ductus arteriosus morphology is crucial in interpreting blood pressure readings taken from such infants, who are usually critically ill. Spontaneous closure of the ductus arteriosus is thought to mediate the frequent observation of sudden clinical deterioration in these infants. It is known that prostaglandin E_1 may be life-saving in such situations by opening the ductus arteriosus and improving flow to the lower body.

DUCTUS ARTERIOSUS IN AORTIC ATRESIA

The entire systemic circulation is dependent on the ductus arteriosus in aortic valve atresia (hypoplastic left-sided heart syndrome). In this situation, as in coarctation of the aorta and interrupted aortic arch, ductal closure leads to severe clinical deterioration. The ductus may not dilate widely and may have residual constriction during pharmacologic manipulation. A widely PDA supplying the

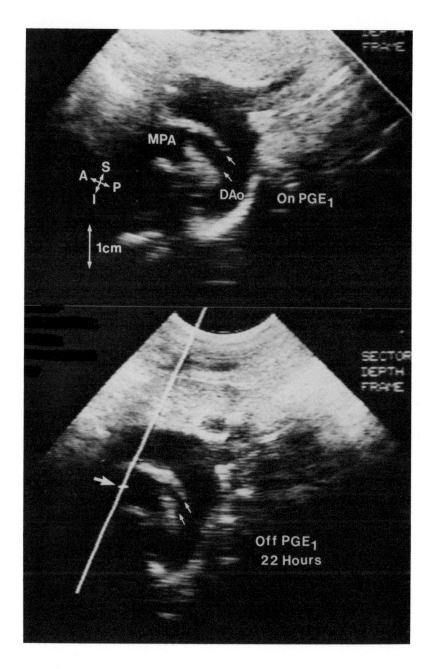

FIG. 8–22. Constriction of the ductus arteriosus in response to prostaglandin E_1 (PGE$_1$) withdrawal. The white arrow shows the sampling site for the left ventricular outflow tract.

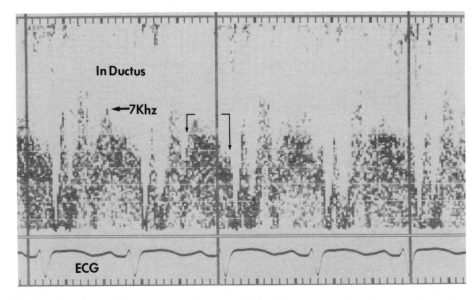

FIG. 8–23. Pulsed Doppler sampling in a PDA with transposition of the great arteries. Note the nearly holodiastolic shunting occurring from the aorta to the main pulmonary artery. 7Khz frequency shift corresponds to 1.1 m/sec velocity across the ductus.

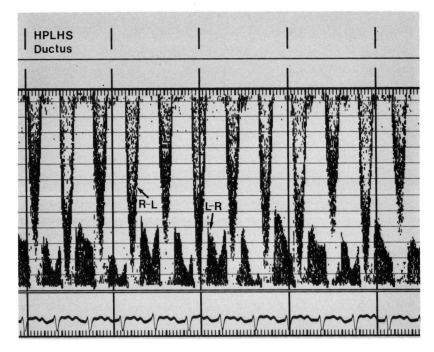

FIG. 8–24. Pulsed Doppler sampling in the ductus arteriosus in a patient with hypoplastic left-sided heart syndrome (HPLHS). There is predominant right-to-left (R–L) shunting followed by a small amount of left-to-right (L–R) shunting in diastole.

hypoplastic ascending aorta can be confirmed by Doppler examination from the suprasternal notch. The bidirectional nature of the flow through the ductus can be assessed by sampling in the midportion of this structure (Figure 8–24).[13]

REFERENCES

1. Smallhorn JF, Huhta JC, Anderson RH, and Macartney FJ: Suprasternal cross-sectional echocardiography in the assessment of patent ductus arteriosus. Br Heart J 48:321, 1982.
2. Sahn DJ, and Allen HD: Real-time cross-sectional echocardiographic imaging and measurement of the patent ductus arteriosus in infants and children. Circulation 58:343, 1978.
3. Huhta JC, Strasburger JF, Carpenter RJ, et al: Pulsed Doppler fetal echocardiography. J Clin Ultrasound 13:247, 1985.
4. Huhta JC, Cohen M, and Gutgesell HP: Patency of the ductus arteriosus in normal neonates: Two-dimensional echocardiography versus Doppler assessment. J Am Coll Cardiol 4:561, 1984.
5. Gentile R, Stevenson G, Dooley T, et al: Pulsed Doppler echocardiographic determination of time of ductal closure in normal newborn infants. J Pediatr 98:443, 1981.
6. McGrath RL, McGuinness GA, Way GL, et al: The silent ductus arteriosus. J Pediatr 93:110, 1978.
7. Valdes-Cruz LM, and Dudell GG: Specificity and accuracy of echocardiographic and clinical criteria for diagnosis of patent ductus arteriosus in fluid-restricted infants. J Pediatr 98:298, 1981.
8. Vick GW, Huhta JC, and Gutgesell HP: Assessment of the ductus arteriosus in preterm infants utilizing suprasternal two-dimensional/Doppler echocardiography. J Am Coll Cardiol 5:973, 1985.
9. Smallhorn JF, Gow R, Olley PM, et al: Combined noninvasive assessment of the patent ductus arteriosus in the preterm infant before and after indomethacin treatment. Am J Cardiol 54:1300, 1984.
10. Huhta JC, Gutgesell HP, Latson LA, and Huffines FD: Two-dimensional echocardiographic assessment of the aorta in infants and children with congenital heart disease. Circulation 70:417, 1984.
11. Huhta JC, Abdallah SA, Nihill MR, and Murphy DJ: The hemodynamic effects of prostaglandin in complete transposition of the great arteries. Presented at the AAP, San Antonio, Oct 1985 (Abstract).
12. Smallhorn JF, Huhta JC, Adams PS, et al: Cross-sectional echocardiographic assessment of coarctation in the sick neonate and infant. Br Heart J 50:349, 1983.
13. Bash SE, Huhta JC, Gutgesell HP, and Ott DA: Echocardiography: Is it accurate enough to guide surgical palliation of hypoplastic left heart syndrome? J Am Coll Cardiol 7:610, 1986.

chapter **9**

PULMONARY ARTERIES

The proximal pulmonary artery confluence can be evaluated by ultrasound techniques. However, because of air in inflated lung parenchyma, the distal pulmonary arteries at the hili of the lungs cannot be imaged. The proximal, intrapericardial pulmonaries, including the *main pulmonary artery* from the heart to the bifurcation, the *right pulmonary artery* from its origin at the bifurcation to slightly beyond the upper lobe branch, and the *left pulmonary artery* from its origin to the point where it crosses in front of the descending aorta, can be seen. This ability to directly visualize the morphology and size of the pulmonaries is extremely useful in the evaluation of children with congenital heart and pulmonary disease. The dimensions and shape of these arteries provide clues to the hemodynamics of the pulmonary circulation and to pulmonary function. In critically ill neonates and children with noncardiac disorders, M-mode and Doppler ultrasonography can be useful in estimating flow and pressure parameters in these vessels.

Ultrasound evaluation of the pulmonary arteries has been described in children using either a parasternal, a subcostal, or a suprasternal ultrasonic window. Limited work has been reported on the quantitation of pulmonary artery size with ultrasound, including normal measurements of the proximal arteries,[1,2] measurements of the right pulmonary artery in tetralogy of Fallot,[3–5] and quantitation of pulmonary artery size in pulmonary atresia.[6,7]

The pulmonary arteries bifurcate from the main pulmonary artery within 2 to

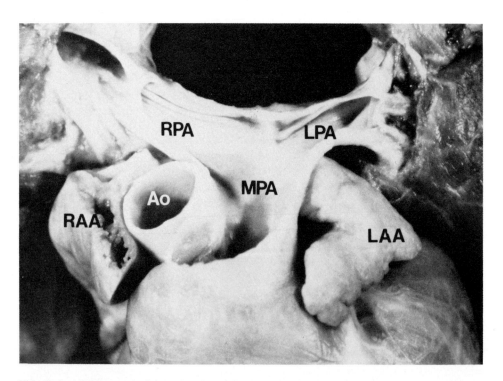

FIG. 9–1. Autopsy specimen showing the bifurcation of the main pulmonary artery (MPA) into the right (RPA) and left pulmonary artery (LPA) branches. Note the course of the right pulmonary artery behind the ascending aorta (Ao), and the position of the atrial appendages (LAA and RAA).

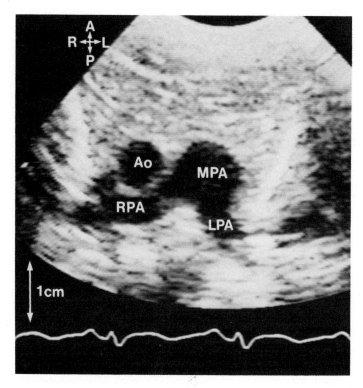

FIG. 9–2. Parasternal imaging of the main pulmonary artery (MPA) with its right and left pulmonary artery branches.

5 cm of the pulmonary valve and right ventricular outflow tract (Figure 9–1) and can be visualized from several approaches, but the suprasternal and parasternal approaches are superior to others. The main pulmonary artery is immediately behind the sternum and can be imaged using both sagittal and coronal scans. From a high left infraclavicular position the length of the main pulmonary artery can be seen (Plate XVIII) in a scan of the right ventricular outflow tract. Transverse parasternal scans show the bifurcation of the main pulmonary artery (Plate XVIV). The right pulmonary artery normally lies in a coronal plane, and a suprasternal scan shows its entire length from its junction with the main artery to the point at which the right superior vena cava crosses it (Plate XX). The left pulmonary artery passes over the left main stem bronchus before its first branch point, while the right pulmonary artery stays anterior to its bronchus. This causes the left pulmonary artery to be a curvilinear structure with an orthogonal orientation with respect to the right pulmonary artery. Therefore the tomographic plane that best cuts the left pulmonary artery is nearly sagittal and is almost at right angles to the imaging plane for the right pulmonary artery (Plate XXI).

NORMAL MORPHOLOGY

MAIN PULMONARY ARTERY

The intrapericardial position of the proximal pulmonaries makes them accessible for ultrasound scanning from midsternal positions. Left parasternal posi-

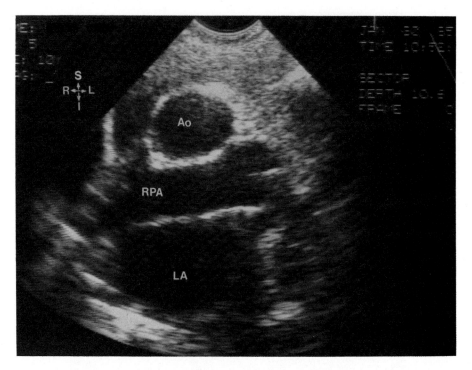

FIG. 9–3. Suprasternal coronal scan showing the aorta (Ao) and the right pulmonary artery (RPA) cut in its long axis. The left atrium is located inferiorly. Note the overlap of the right superior vena cava to the right of the aorta and the right pulmonary artery.

tions, especially immediately below the suprasternal notch, are valuable in the neonate and can be used in the older child placed in the left lateral position. The main pulmonary artery is normally a tubular structure with only mild dilation after its origin from the heart. From this approach the flow velocity in the main pulmonary artery and immediately above the valve can be measured by Doppler ultrasonography (see Figure 3–8). The angle of the Doppler beam to the flow of blood usually is greater than 30 degrees, and the subcostal approach where a better angle can be obtained is preferable.

The size of the main pulmonary artery is usually about 10 to 15% greater than the semilunar valve anulus from which it arises and is normally about 30% larger than either branch. Significant departure from this relationship is a clue to congenital heart disease (see further on).

The normal main pulmonary artery courses posteriorly and superiorly to its bifurcation toward the lungs. Because this bifurcation is a frequent site of stenosis, it should be examined routinely. This can be done from scans approximately 45 degrees from the transverse plane; its normal appearance is that of "trousers," with the legs being the pulmonary arteries (Figure 9–2).

RIGHT PULMONARY ARTERY

The proximal right pulmonary artery can be seen from the subcostal position, however the suprasternal position allows imaging at right angles to this structure

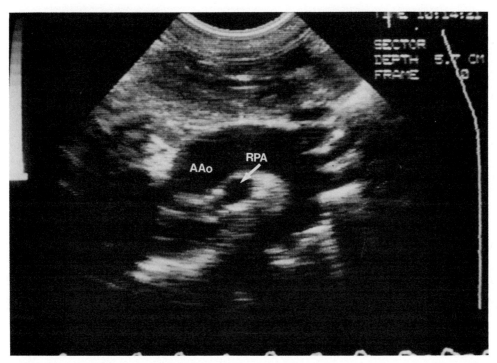

FIG. 9–4. Sagittal scanning of the normal ascending aorta. The right pulmonary artery (RPA) is seen in cross-section as a circular structure immediately behind the ascending aorta (Aao).

and visualization as distal as the right upper lobe branch in nearly every patient (Figure 9–3). Orthogonal to this scan, the right pulmonary artery is seen in cross-section immediately behind the ascending aorta (Figure 9–4). When there is marked right pulmonary artery dilation, sagittal scans to the right of the spine may cut both the lower and upper branches. Pulmonary artery sizes can be measured as shown in Figure 9–5. The right pulmonary artery runs in front of its accompanying bronchus, giving it a relatively direct course to the hilus compared with the left pulmonary artery.

LEFT PULMONARY ARTERY

The left pulmonary artery lies in a plane similar to that of the ductus arteriosus (see Chapter 7) and can be imaged from sagittal scans high on the chest. After spontaneous closure of the ductus arteriosus with normal obliteration of the pulmonary diverticulum of the ductus, the left pulmonary branch orifice may be narrowed, causing proximal pulmonary artery stenosis. This may result from extension of ductus tissue onto the pulmonary artery and postnatal constriction. Such a discrete narrowing may be a cause of an innocent heart murmur, which resembles that of a PDA in the newborn period. Utilizing pulsed Doppler methods, this can be confirmed by withdrawing the sample volume from the distal left to the main pulmonary artery (Figure 9–6).

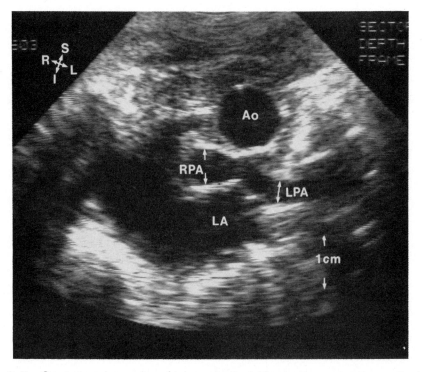

FIG. 9–5. Suprasternal scanning of a hypoplastic right pulmonary artery in a patient with severe pulmonary stenosis and cyanosis. Note the right pulmonary artery behind the dilated aorta and its origination from the main pulmonary artery.

ABNORMALITIES

DILATION

Dilation of the pulmonary arterial tree may be caused by (1) stenosis, (2) increased pulmonary blood flow, or (3) severe elevation of pulmonary artery pressure (pulmonary hypertension).

The most common cause of dilation of the main pulmonary artery only is turbulence from pulmonary valve *stenosis*. The energy released distal to a severe obstruction to flow causes enlargement of the artery where the jet hits the arterial wall. The degree of so-called poststenotic dilation correlates roughly with the severity of the stenosis. Typically, the main pulmonary artery in pulmonary stenosis is dilated, while the proximal left and right arteries are close to normal thickness. Such poststenotic dilation occurs downstream to congenital or acquired discrete narrowing of either the main or branch pulmonary arteries.

Increased pulmonary blood flow in excess of normal results in dilation of the pulmonary arteries in order to accommodate the increased stroke volume ejected into them. Enlargement of the main, left, and right pulmonary arteries may

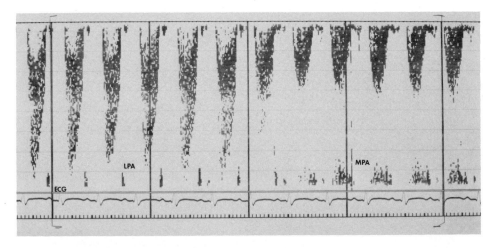

FIG. 9–6.   Doppler sampling in the distal left pulmonary artery and withdrawal of the sample volume into the main pulmonary artery. Increased Doppler blood flow velocity distal to mild proximal left pulmonary artery stenosis is shown.

occur with (1) pulmonary artery pressure higher than normal, as in ventricular septal defect, or (2) high flow with normal pressure, as in atrial septal defect (Figure 9–7). Increased stroke volume may also result from pulmonary insufficiency causing enlargement of the proximal arteries, as is often seen after transanular patch enlargement of the right ventricular outflow tract to relieve stenosis.

When severe and end-stage *pulmonary hypertension* is present, the proximal pulmonary arteries are enlarged and quickly taper near the lung hilus. Pulmonary insufficiency may contribute to arterial enlargement in such cases, as it is almost invariably present. Work using Doppler methods to quantitate pulmonary pressure and flow in these situations is preliminary but promises to be useful clinically and provide new information concerning the hemodynamic changes that accompany increasing pulmonary vascular resistance.[8–10]

A poorly understood etiology for massive dilation of the proximal pulmonary arteries is *absent pulmonary valve syndrome*. This syndrome is associated with huge pulmonary arteries sometimes three or four times the size of the aorta (Figure 9–8), and pulmonary anular constriction and fibrosis result in stenosis and insufficiency.[11] The severe arterial dilation frequently progresses to cause compression of the bronchi and respiratory failure in infancy.

HYPOPLASIA

The final common pathway of pulmonary artery hypoplasia is *decreased pulmonary blood flow*. Flow may be reduced because of (1) decreased cross-sectional area of the pulmonary vascular bed, (2) obstruction to pulmonary venous return, or (3) right ventricular outflow tract obstruction. A decreased pulmonary bed

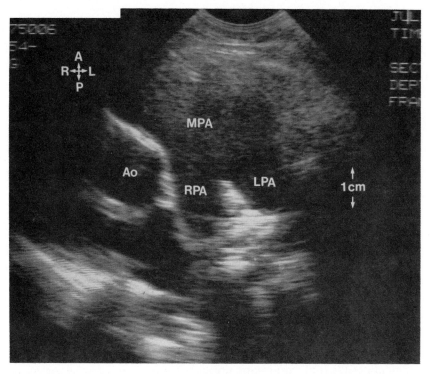

FIG. 9–7. Parasternal scan of a dilated main pulmonary artery (MPA) attributable to a large left-to-right shunt. Note the dilated right and left pulmonary artery branches as well.

may be caused by lung hypoplasia or lung damage. Pulmonary artery hypoplasia due to pulmonary venous obstruction is discussed in Chapter 10.

Right ventricular outflow tract obstruction, when severe and associated with ventricular septal defect or atrial septal defect, results in shunting of blood away from the pulmonary circulation via either of these defects. The resulting decrease in pulmonary blood flow leads directly to underdevelopment of the pulmonary arterial bed and to smaller than normal size of the pulmonary arteries. This hypoplasia may occur because of poor flow in utero or rarely may be related to abnormal arterial wall development (Figure 9–9).

Confident identification of the left and right pulmonary arteries and correct diagnosis of the sources of pulmonary blood supply by ultrasound imaging are the basis for palliative surgery in cyanotic neonates without cardiac catheterization. Abnormalities such as tetralogy of Fallot, pulmonary atresia, and Ebstein's malformation of the tricuspid valve manifest hypoplasia of the pulmonary arteries and are all examples of right-sided heart obstruction that leads to right-to-left intracardiac shunt. In some types of congenital heart disease the size of the pulmonary arteries will determine the most appropriate type of surgery. Following an intervention to enlarge the arteries, cross-sectional ultrasound imaging is useful to measure the artery size.

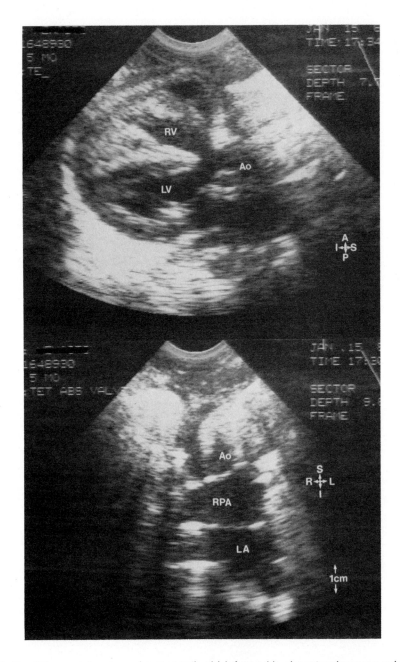

FIG. 9–8. Ultrasound scans of a 5-month-old infant with absent pulmonary valve syndrome. The ventricular anatomy is typical of tetralogy of Fallot (upper panel), with an overriding aorta. Suprasternal coronal scans (lower panel) show a markedly dilated right pulmonary artery twice the size of the aorta above it.

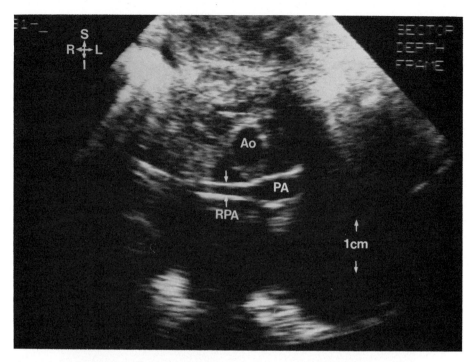

FIG. 9–9. Hypoplasia of the right pulmonary artery seen from suprasternal scans in a critically ill newborn. Severe pulmonary artery hypoplasia was related to lung hypoplasia and pulmonary atresia with intact septum.

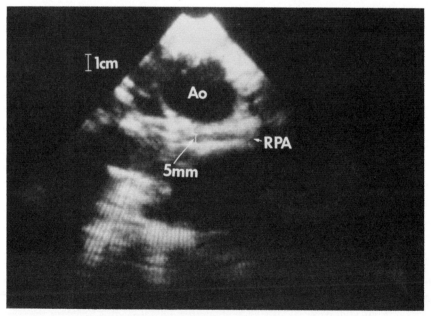

FIG. 9–10. Hypoplastic right pulmonary artery measuring 5 mm in diameter on suprasternal scans in a patient with pulmonary atresia and ventricular septal defect.

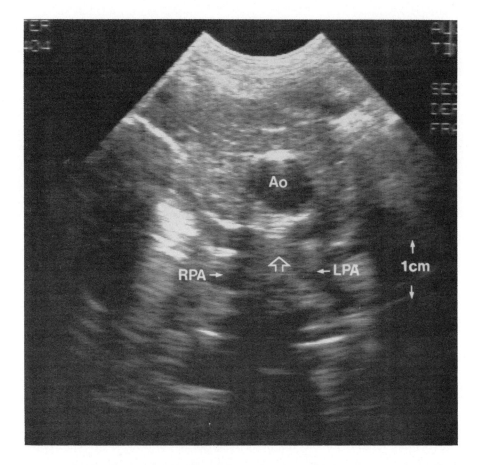

FIG. 9–11. Nonconfluent pulmonary arteries in a patient with a left and right patent ductus arteriosus and pulmonary atresia. Note the absence of a main pulmonary artery (open white arrow).

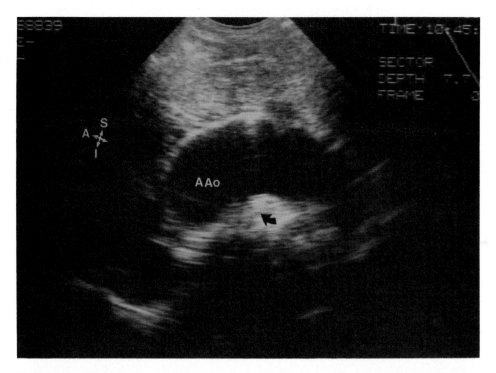

FIG. 9–12. Parasternal scan of the ascending aorta demonstrating marked dilation and no evidence of a right pulmonary artery posterior to it. This patient had nonconfluent pulmonary arteries.

PULMONARY ATRESIA

Pulmonary blood supply in pulmonary atresia may be *unifocal*[12] from a ductus arteriosus or *multifocal* from major aortopulmonary collateral arteries. Cross-sectional ultrasonography is useful in identifying the presence of intrapericardial, confluent pulmonary arteries in the midline of the thorax.[7] These arteries may be very small (2 to 3 mm in diameter) (Figure 9–10) and in unusual patients may only be fibrous strands. In such children the collateral arteries may be identified by their more posterior position in the chest. Angiography is needed to define the blood supply and distal connections of each lung segment.

ABNORMAL ORIGIN

The right or left pulmonary artery may originate from the ascending aorta as a congenital abnormality (see Chapter 5). In such cases it is important to define the site of origin of the artery, and this can be accomplished by transverse and sagittal scans.[13] The origin of the pulmonary artery in the truncus arteriosus can also be defined accurately by cross-sectional ultrasound imaging (see Chapter 2).

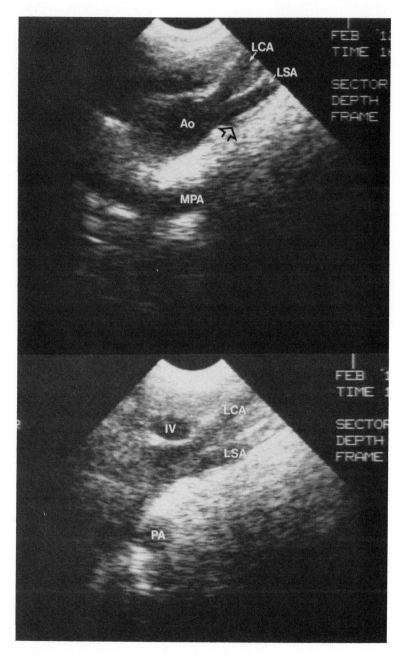

FIG. 9–13. Suprasternal scans toward the left shoulder of a right aortic arch with mirror image branching and a small occluded left ductus arteriosus (open black arrow in upper panel). There was no evidence of a left pulmonary artery connecting to the main pulmonary artery (lower panel). This condition has been termed "absent left pulmonary artery." Ao = aorta, IV = innominate vein, LSA = left subclavian artery, MPA-PA = main pulmonary artery.

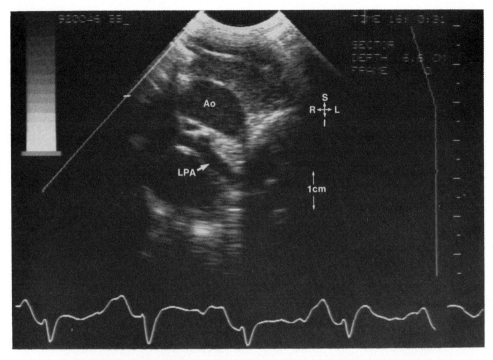

FIG. 9–14.   Imaging of a hypoplastic left pulmonary artery in pulmonary atresia in a cyanotic newborn infant. The scan is sagittal and anterior to the left ductus arteriosus, which was supplying these confluent pulmonary arteries.

Rarely the left or right pulmonary artery may arise separately from a ductus arteriosus. On the side of the aortic arch this is usually a typical origin under the arch (see Chapter 8), but on the side opposite the arch the ductus and pulmonary artery arise from the innominate artery. If the right and left pulmonary arteries are nonconfluent, then either or both may originate from a ductus arteriosus (Figures 9–11 and 9–12). In such cases and in some cases of hypoplastic pulmonary arteries with pulmonary atresia, there is atresia of the main pulmonary artery as well as of the pulmonary valve. After ductus closure, a pulmonary artery arising from it may not be supplied with blood (Figure 9–13).

The left pulmonary artery may be difficult to image in pulmonary atresia. This vessel is oriented in a sagittal plane and can be seen during ductus examination (Figure 9–14).

ACQUIRED ABNORMALITIES

The pulmonary artery branches may be abnormal but only their proximal portions may be examined by ultrasonography.[14]

Stenosis of the pulmonary arteries may be congenital; however, it is commonly due to previous surgery. Aortopulmonary artery shunts used for palliation of

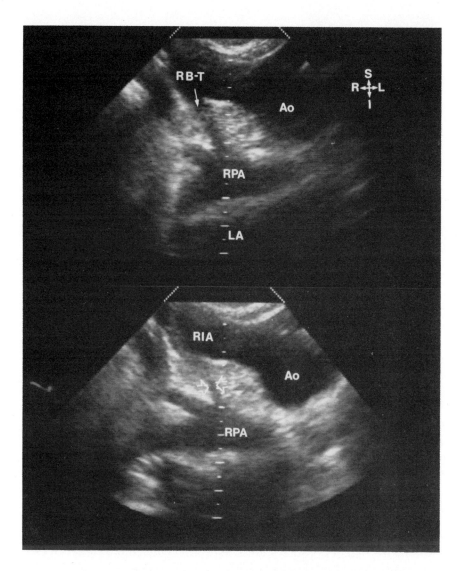

FIG. 9–15. Imaging of a right Blalock-Taussig shunt from the suprasternal approach. A coronal scan visualizes the right innominate artery and the origin of the right subclavian artery, which has been turned down and anastomosed to the right pulmonary artery (upper panel). The entry of the shunt into the pulmonary artery near the origin of the right upper lobe of the right pulmonary artery is well visualized (open white arrows, lower panel).

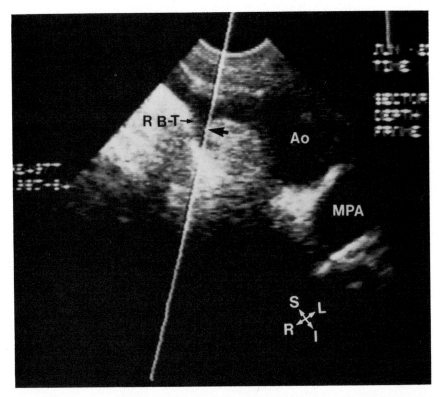

FIG. 9–16. Illustration of the technique for determination of shunt patency using Doppler echocardiography. The origin of the right Blalock-Taussig anastomosis is imaged from a suprasternal scan, and the sample volume position (black arrow) is oriented in the shunt.

cyanotic congenital heart disease may lead to mild or severe narrowing of the pulmonary arteries. The ascending aorta to right pulmonary artery anastomosis is likely to cause this complication,[15] but any type of anastomosis may cause this. At Texas Children's Hospital we have used cross-sectional ultrasonography routinely for the evaluation of systemic-to-pulmonary shunts and their effects on hypoplastic pulmonary arteries (Figure 9–15). Doppler ultrasound is useful in assessing the patency of such shunts, especially when there are several sources of pulmonary blood flow (Figure 9–16).[16,17] Continuous wave Doppler technique may be a useful adjunct to the measurement of the pulmonary artery pressure distal to such a shunt (Figure 9–17).

Banding of the pulmonary artery is a palliative operation performed to decrease the pulmonary blood flow and pressure when intracardiac surgical repair is not feasible. The constriction produced by a pulmonary artery band can be assessed by cross-sectional ultrasound imaging (Figure 9–18). Continuous wave Doppler ultrasound can be used to measure the blood flow velocity across such a constriction.[18] Then the modified Bernouilli equation can be used to calculate the gradient. It is known that a main pulmonary band may migrate in the months

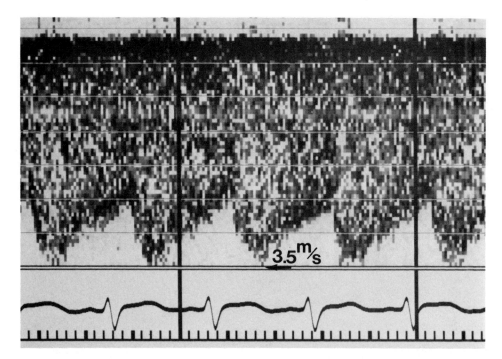

FIG. 9–17. Continuous wave Doppler in a right Blalock-Taussig shunt. Note the continuous pattern of blood flow inferiorly through the shunt and the relatively high systolic and diastolic velocities.

following the surgery and kink one pulmonary artery. This complication can be detected by ultrasonic scans of the pulmonary artery confluence from the chest and suprasternal notch.

Aneurysmal dilation of the main pulmonary artery may result from a systemic-to-pulmonary artery shunt.[19]

An extracardiac conduit may be used to treat complex congenital heart disease, and Doppler techniques are useful to detect and quantitate obstruction.[20]

CORONARY ARTERY ORIGIN FROM A PULMONARY ARTERY

Ultrasonic imaging and Doppler techniques have been used successfully to diagnose anomalous origin of a coronary artery from the pulmonary tree.[21–23] Detection of antegrade diastolic flow velocity in the main pulmonary artery is useful in this condition (Figure 9–19).[24] However, false negative findings are possible, and angiography still is the procedure of choice when this diagnosis is suspected.

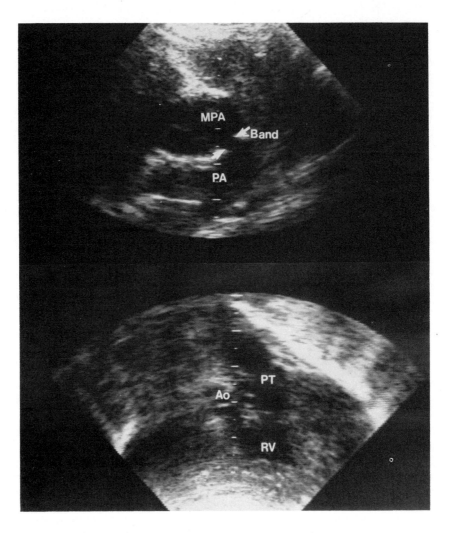

FIG. 9–18. Parasternal imaging of a pulmonary artery band that is constricting the pulmonary artery in its midportion (upper panel). This patient had double-outlet right ventricle, with the pulmonary trunk to the left and the aorta to the right (lower panel).

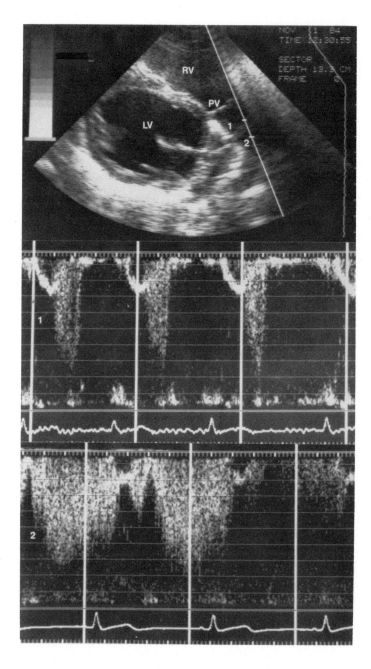

FIG. 9–19. Doppler sampling in a patient with anomalous origin of the right coronary artery from the main pulmonary trunk. The Doppler sample volume is positioned immediately above the pulmonary valve (1) and shows a late diastolic antegrade turbulence superimposed on normal antegrade pulmonary valve flow. More distal sampling in the main pulmonary artery (2) shows nearly holodiastolic antegrade turbulence.

REFERENCES

1. Snider AR, Enderlein MA, Teitel DF and Juster RP: Two-dimensional echocardiographic determination of aortic and pulmonary artery sizes from infancy to adulthood in normal subjects. Am J Cardiol 53:218, 1984.
2. Allen HD, Goldberg SJ, Sahn DJ, et al: Suprasternal notch echocardiography: Assessment of its clinical utility in pediatric cardiology. Circulation 55:605, 1977.
3. Lappen RS, Riggs TW, Lapin GD, et al: Two-dimensional echocardiographic measurement of right pulmonary artery diameter in infants and children. J Am Coll Cardiol 2:121, 1983.
4. Cloez JL, Hda A, Brunotte F, et al: [Evaluation of the pulmonary artery and its branches by two-dimensional echocardiography in the tetralogy of Fallot and pulmonary atresia in infants. Angiocardiographic correlation and therapeutic implications]. Arch Fr Pediatr 41:307, 1984.
5. Allen HD, Sahn DJ, Lange L, and Goldberg SJ: Noninvasive assessment of surgical systemic to pulmonary artery shunts by range-gated pulsed Doppler echocardiography. J Pediatr 94:395, 1979.
6. Gutgesell HP, Huhta JC, Cohen MH, and Latson LA: Two-dimensional echocardiographic assessment of pulmonary artery and aortic arch anatomy in cyanotic infants. J Am Coll Cardiol 4:1242, 1984.
7. Huhta JC, Piehler JM, Tajik AJ, et al: Two-dimensional echocardiographic detection and measurement of the right pulmonary artery in pulmonary atresia-ventricular septal defect: Angiographic and surgical correlation. Am J Cardiol 49:1235, 1982.
8. Kosturakis D, Goldberg S, Allen H, et al: Doppler echocardiographic prediction of pulmonary arterial hypertension in congenital heart disease. Am J Cardiol 53:1110, 1984.
9. Hatle L, Angelsen BA, and Tromsdal A: Non-invasive estimation of pulmonary artery systolic pressure with Doppler ultrasound. Br Heart J 45:157, 1981.
10. Stevenson JG, Kawabori I, and Guntheroth WG: Noninvasive estimation of peak pulmonary artery pressure by M-mode echocardiography. J Am Coll Cardiol 4:1021, 1984.
11. Cheatham JP, Latson LA, and Gutgesell HP: Echocardiographic pulsed Doppler features of absent pulmonary valve syndrome in the neonate. Am J Cardiol 49:1773, 1982.
12. Faller K, Haworth SG, Taylor JFN, and Macartney FJ: Duplicate sources of pulmonary blood supply in pulmonary atresia with ventricular septal defect. Br Heart J 46:253, 1981.
13. Smallhorn JF, Anderson RH, and Macartney FJ: Two-dimensional echocardiographic assessment of communications between ascending aorta and pulmonary trunk or individual pulmonary arteries. Br Heart J 47:563, 1982.
14. Piot JD, Rey C, Leriche H, et al: [Assessment of the branches of the pulmonary artery by 2-dimensional echocardiography.] Arch Mal Coeur 76:530, 1983.
15. Tay DJ, Engle MA, Ehlers KH, and Levin AR: Early results and late developments of the Waterston anastomosis. Circulation 50:220, 1974.
16. Stevenson JG, Kawabori I, and Bailey WW: Noninvasive evaluation of Blalock-Taussig shunts: Determination of patency and differentiation from patent ductus arteriosus by Doppler echocardiography. Am Heart J 106:1121, 1983.
17. Allen HD, Sahn DJ, Lange L, and Goldberg SJ: Noninvasive assessment of surgical systemic to pulmonary artery shunts by range-gated pulsed Doppler echocardiography. J Pediatr 94:395, 1979.
18. Fyfe DA, Currie PJ, Seward JB, et al: Continuous-wave Doppler determination of the pressure gradient across pulmonary artery bands: Hemodynamic correlation in 20 patients. Mayo Clin Proc 59:744, 1984.
19. Lakhani ZM, McGarry KM, Taylor RF, et al: Two-dimensional echocardiographic detection of left pulmonary artery aneurysm following Potts' anastomosis. Chest 84:782, 1983.
20. Reeder GS, Currie PJ, Fyfe DA, et al: Extracardiac conduit obstruction: Initial experience in the use of Doppler echocardiography for noninvasive estimation of pressure gradient. J Am Coll Cardiol 4:1006, 1984.
21. Fisher EA, Sepehri B, Lendrum B, et al: Two-dimensional echocardiographic visualization of the left coronary artery in anomalous origin of the left coronary artery from the pulmonary artery. Pre- and postoperative studies. Circulation 63:698, 1981.
22. Terai M, Nagai Y, and Toba T: Cross-sectional echocardiographic findings of anomalous origin of left coronary artery from pulmonary artery. Br Heart J 50:104, 1983.
23. Worsham C, Sanders SP, and Burger BM: Origin of the right coronary artery from the pulmonary trunk: Diagnosis by two-dimensional echocardiography. Am J Cardiol 55:232, 1985.
24. King DH, Danford DA, Huhta JC, and Gutgesell HP: Noninvasive detection of anomalous origin of the left main coronary artery from the pulmonary trunk by pulsed Doppler echocardiography. (Brief Report). Am J Cardiol 55:608, 1985.

COLOR PLATES

PLATE I

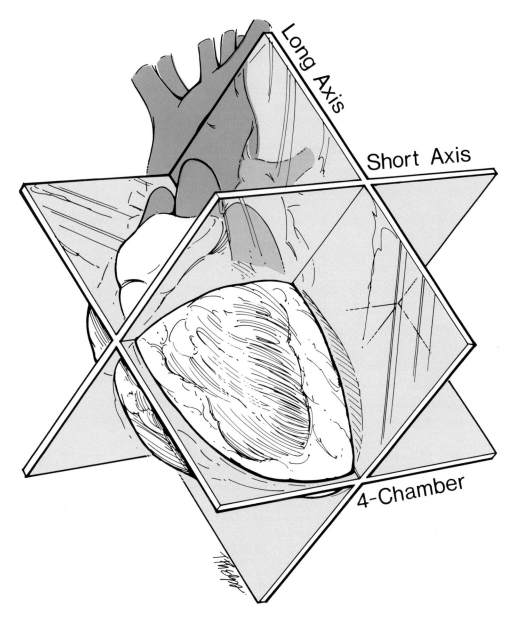

Standardized planes for examination of the heart by cardiac ultrasonography. Note that the cardiac-oriented planes are not related to the standardized sagittal, transverse, and coronal radiographic planes in any predictable fashion.

PLATE II

TRANSVERSE SCANS

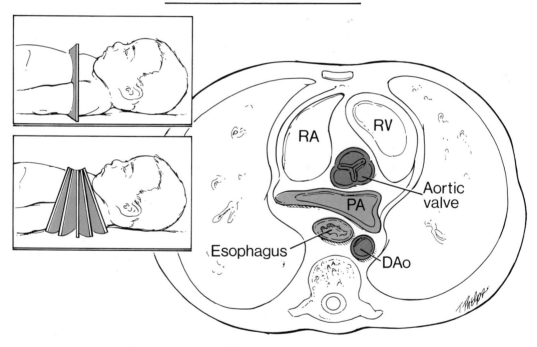

Transverse images of the chest are displayed as if the observer were sitting at the patient's feet and looking toward the head. Cross-sectional ultrasonic scans may vary slightly from the standardized transverse images obtainable by other methods (compare the two insets). DAo = descending aorta, PA = pulmonary artery, RA = right atrium, RV = right ventricle.

PLATE III

SAGITTAL SCANS

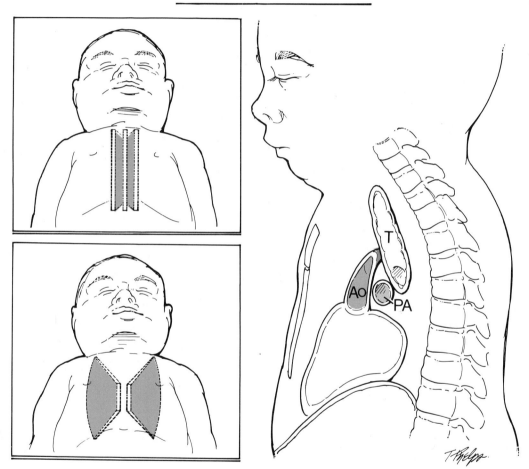

Sagittal sector ultrasound scans of the chest must originate near the parasternal region because of the limitations of ultrasonic windows (see Chapter 1). These appear similar to the standard radiographic sagittal plants obtained by other methods (compare the two insets).

PLATE IV

CORONAL SCANS

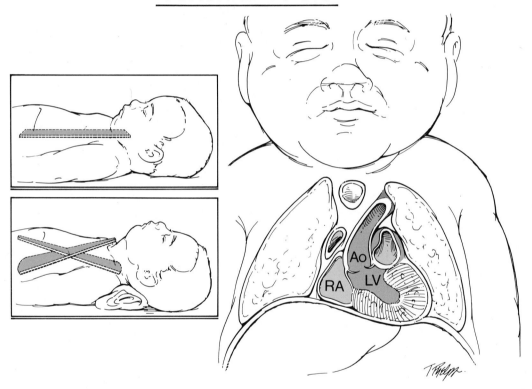

Technique of coronal scans either from the suprasternal notch or the subcostal region. The ultrasonic scans approximate but are not exactly the same as those by other tomographic techniques (compare the two insets).

PLATE V

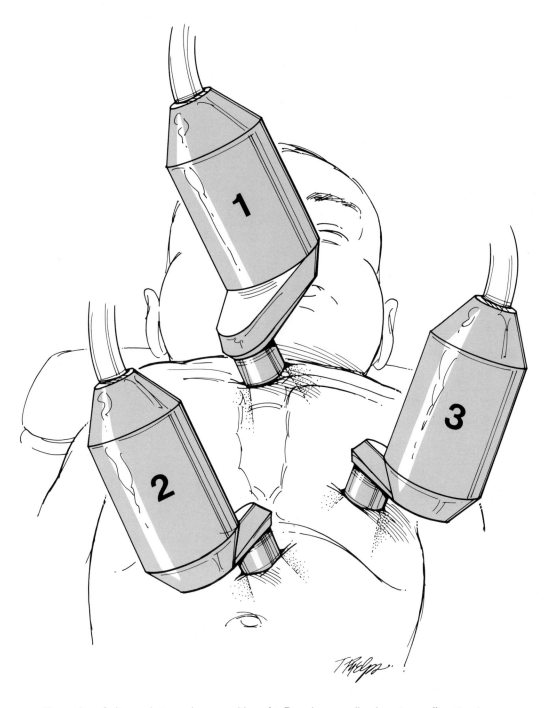

Examples of ultrasonic transducer positions for Doppler sampling in extracardiac structures. The suprasternal (1), the subcostal (2), and the apical (3) approaches are used in a complementary fashion to obtain satisfactory sampling angles in each structure.

PLATE VI

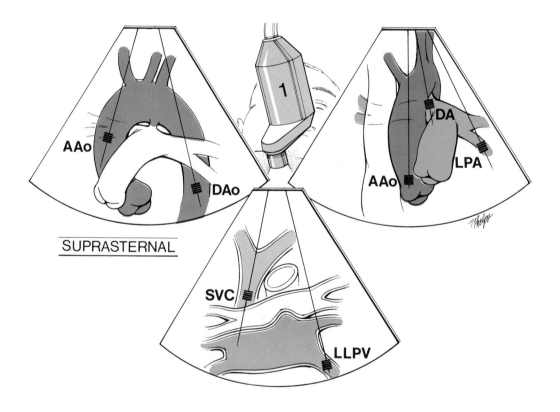

SUPRASTERNAL

Doppler sampling from the suprasternal projection. Sampling is possible in the ascending aorta (AAo), descending aorta (DAo), ductus arterious (DA), left pulmonary artery (LPA), superior vena cava (SVC), and left lower pulmonary vein (LLPV).

PLATE VII

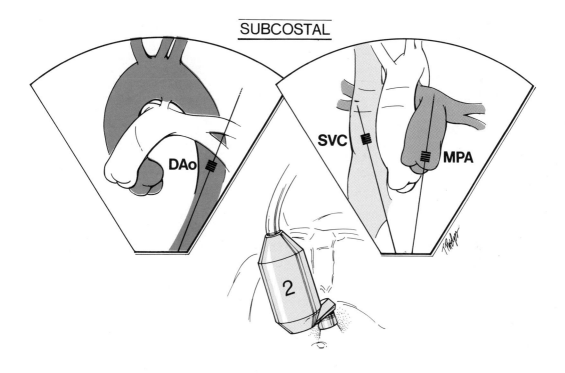

SUBCOSTAL

Doppler sampling from the subcostal approach. Sampling is useful clinically in the descending aorta (DAo), the superior vena cava (SVC), and an optimal angle is obtained at the pulmonary valve of the pattern in the main pulmonary artery (MPA).

PLATE VIII

APICAL

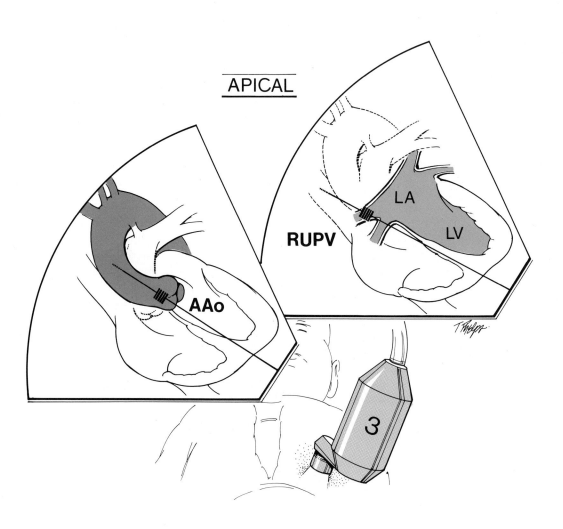

Apical Doppler sampling techniques with the sample volume placed in the ascending aorta (AAo) and the right upper pulmonary vein (RUPV).

PLATE IX

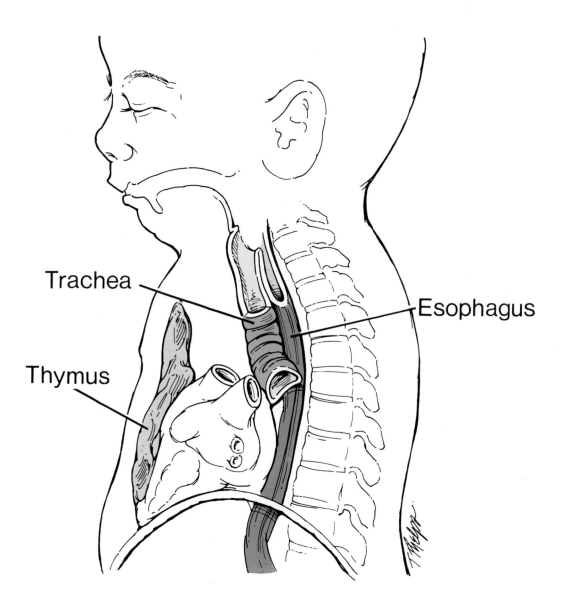

Trachea

Esophagus

Thymus

Composite drawing illustrating the locations of the thymus, the trachea, and the esophagus in a child.

PLATE X

RIGHT

LEFT

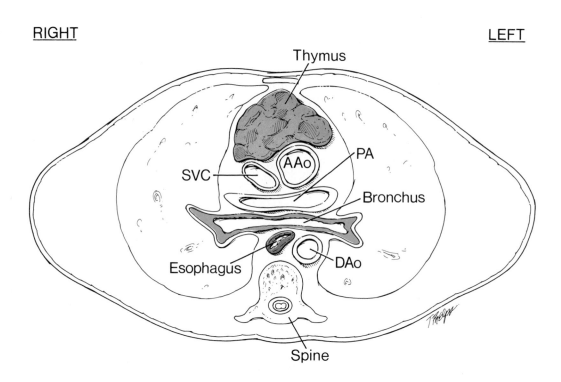

Transverse plane showing the orientation of the thymus, trachea, and esophagus with respect to the pulmonary arteries and aorta. AAo = ascending aorta, DAo = descending aorta, PA = pulmonary artery, (SVC) = superior vena cava.

PLATE XI

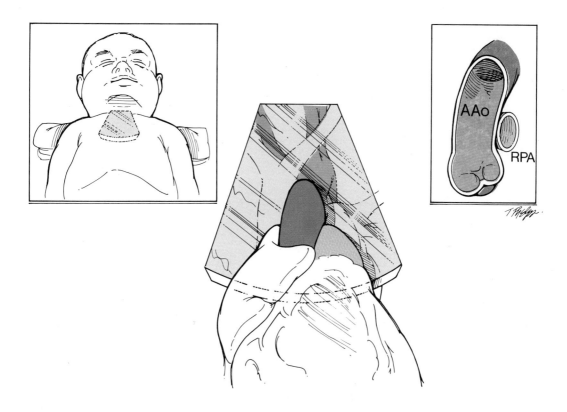

Technique of suprasternal imaging of the origin of the ascending aorta (AAo) and its intra-pericardial course immediately above the aortic valve. The transducer is oriented in a nearly coronal plane.

PLATE XII

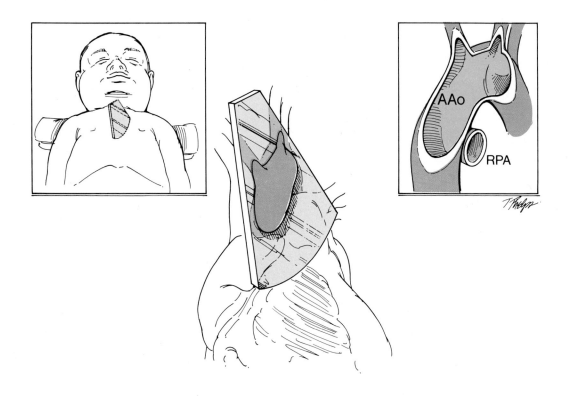

Imaging technique for the ascending aorta (AAo). The upper portion of the ascending aorta, from its supravalvar region to the origin of the brachiocephalic arteries, is seen by placing the transducer in the suprasternal notch and rotating counterclockwise.

PLATE XIII

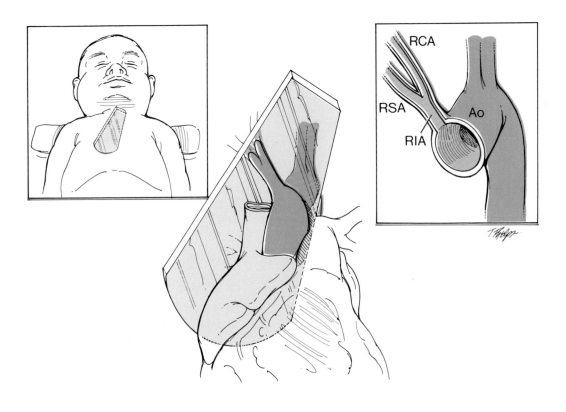

Technique of ultrasound examination of the origin of the right innominate artery from the aortic arch (Ao). Note the plane directed toward the right shoulder from the suprasternal notch transecting the origin of the right innominate artery (RIA) from the aortic arch. The innominate artery branches into the right carotid (RCA) and the right subclavian arteries (RSA).

PLATE XIV

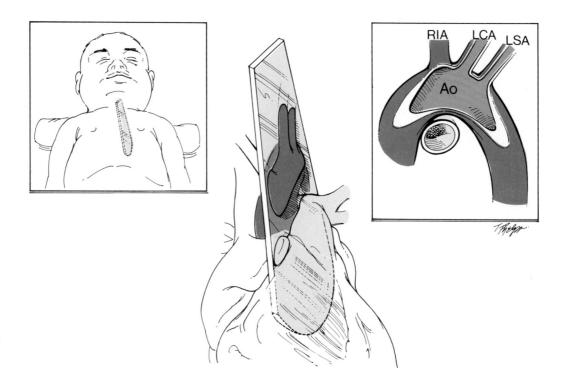

Technique of ultrasound imaging of the brachiocephalic vessels from the suprasternal notch. With a slight counterclockwise rotation of the transducer, the left carotid (LCA) and left subclavian arteries (LSA) are seen to originate from the aortic arch (Ao) in a plane obtained from the suprasternal notch.

PLATE XV

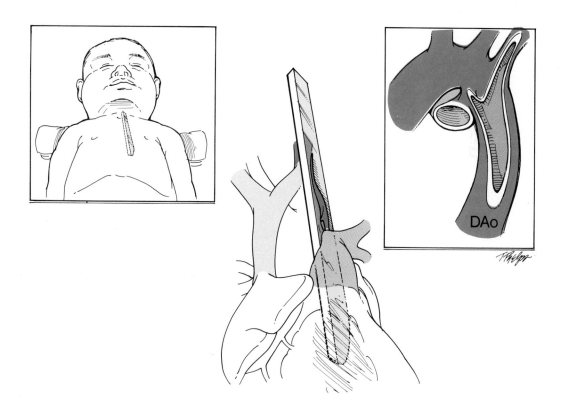

Technique of ultrasound imaging of the aortic isthmus and upper descending aorta in sagittal scans from the suprasternal approach. From the suprasternal notch the ultrasound beam is oriented sagittally, scanning slightly to the left.

PLATE XVI

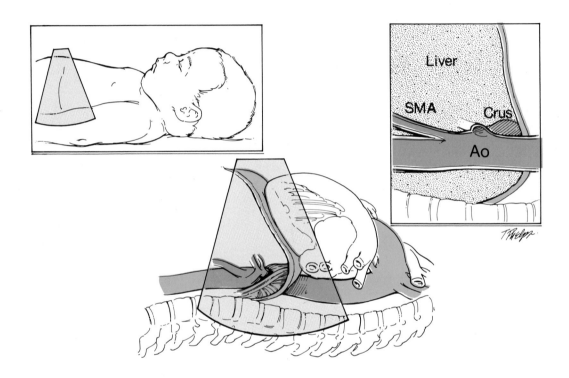

Technique of ultrasound scanning of the thoracic and abdominal portions of the descending aorta. SMA = superior mesentric artery, Crus = crus of the diaphragm, Ao = Aorta.

PLATE XVII

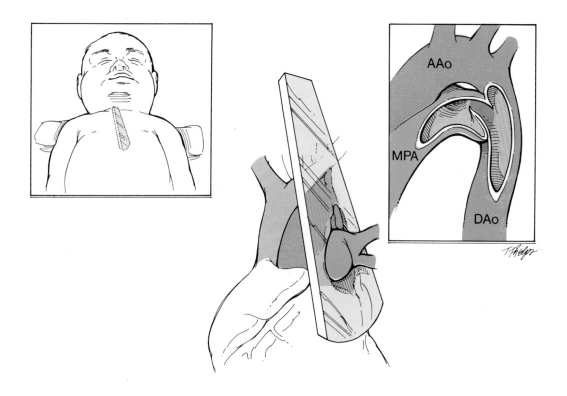

The technique of imaging the ductus arteriosus. The ultrasonic scan is directed from the suprasternal notch or the right neck toward the left and anterior. AAo = ascending aorta, DAo = descending aorta, MPA = main pulmonary artery.

PLATE XVIII

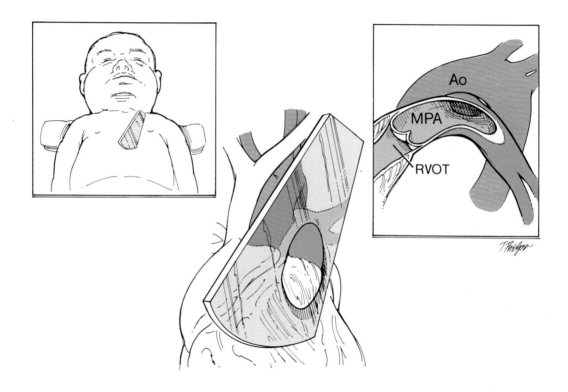

Illustration of the technique of scanning the right ventricular outflow tract (RVOT) and proximal main pulmonary artery (MPA).

PLATE XIX

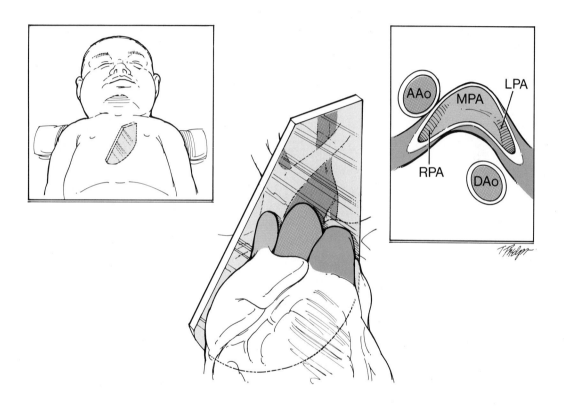

Technique of scanning the main pulmonary trunk and its pulmonary artery branches. AAo = ascending aorta, DAo = descending aorta, LPA = left pulmonary artery, MPA = main pulmonary artery, RPA = right pulmonary artery.

PLATE XX

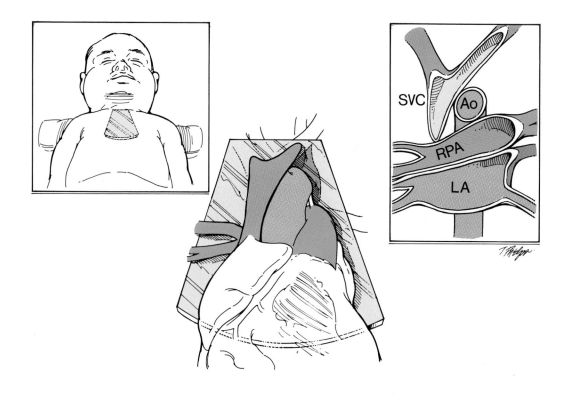

Technique of right pulmonary artery examination from the suprasternal notch from its origin at the main pulmonary artery to the region of right upper pulmonary artery branching. Ao = aorta, LA = left atrium, RPA = right pulmonary artery, SVC = superior vena cava.

PLATE XXI

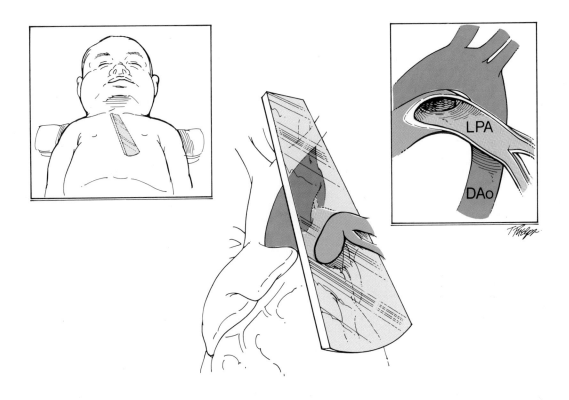

Technique of scanning the left pulmonary artery with the transducer slightly anterior to the scans for the ductus arteriosus visualization (compare with PLATE XVII). LPA = left pulmonary artery, DAo = descending aorta.

PLATE XXII

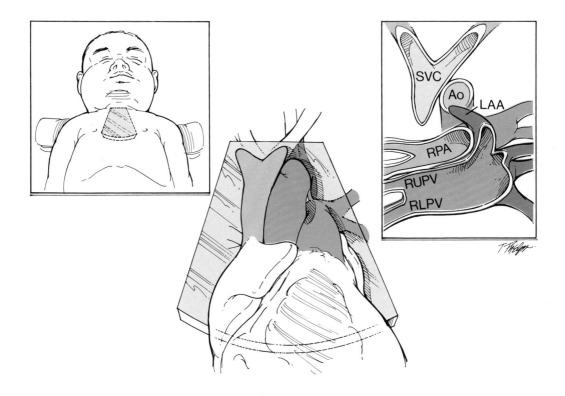

Technique of imaging the right upper (RUPV) and right lower pulmonary veins (RLPV) from suprasternal scans. Note that the origin of the left atrial appendage (LAA) can also be seen in this projection.

PLATE XXIII

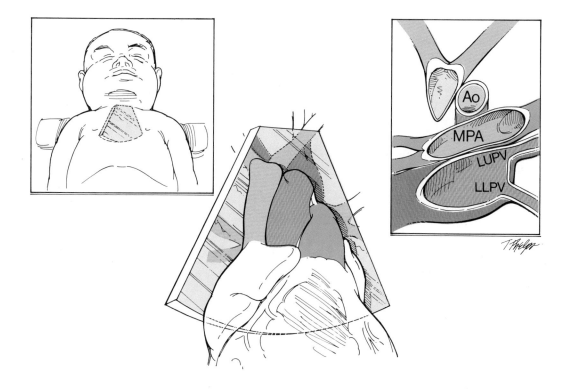

Technique of suprasternal imaging of the left pulmonary veins. Note the left upper (LUPV) and left lower pulmonary veins (LLPV) entering the left atrium. This scan is obtained with slight counterclockwise rotation of the transducer in the suprasternal notch from the position of Plate XVII. Ao = aorta, MPA = main pulmonary artery.

PLATE XXIV

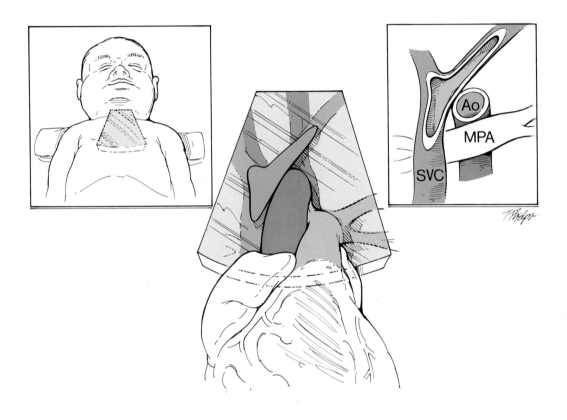

Technique of suprasternal scans for imaging of the innominate vein and upper portion of the superior vena cava. The transducer is placed in the suprasternal notch to obtain a coronal scan. Ao = aorta, MPA = main pulmonary artery, SVC = superior vena cava.

PLATE XXV

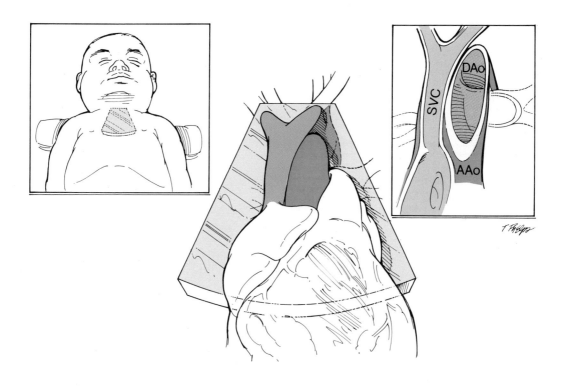

Technique of suprasternal scanning of the right superior vena cava (SVC) with slight anterior scanning as compared with Plate XXIV.

PLATE XXVI

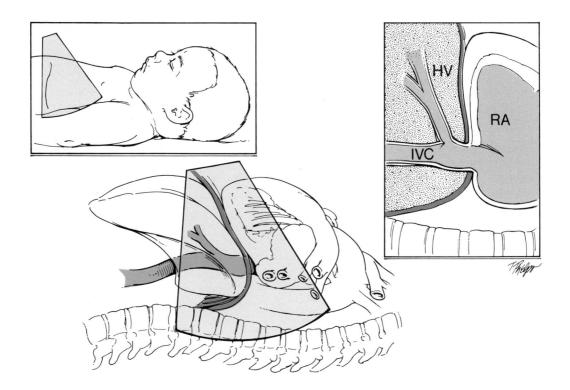

Technique of imaging of the inferior vena cava (IVC) and hepatic veins (HV) using subcostal sagittal scans.

PLATE XXVII

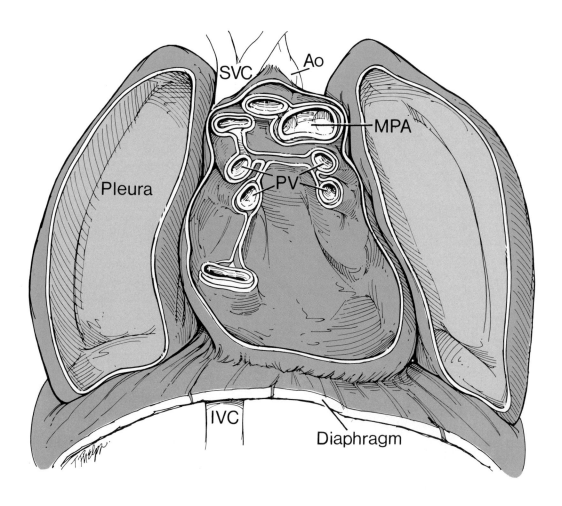

Schematic drawing showing the pleural and pericardial reflections with the heart and lungs removed. The vascular structures entering the pericardium, including the pulmonary veins (PV), superior (SVC) and inferior venae cavae (IVC), and aorta (Ao) and main pulmonary arteries (MPA) are all enveloped by pericardium. The parietal pleura surrounds the lungs and reflects onto the pericardium. The pericardial diaphragmatic reflection is also illustrated.

PLATE XXVIII

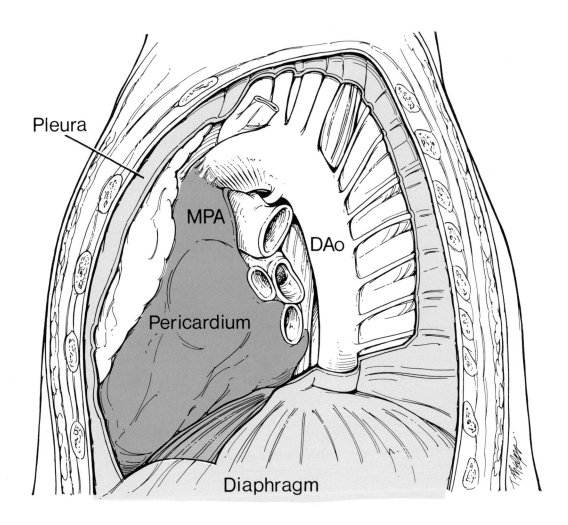

Sagittal scan illustrating the parietal pleura and pericardium and its reflection from the ascending aorta and main pulmonary trunk. DAo = descending aorta.

PLATE XXIX

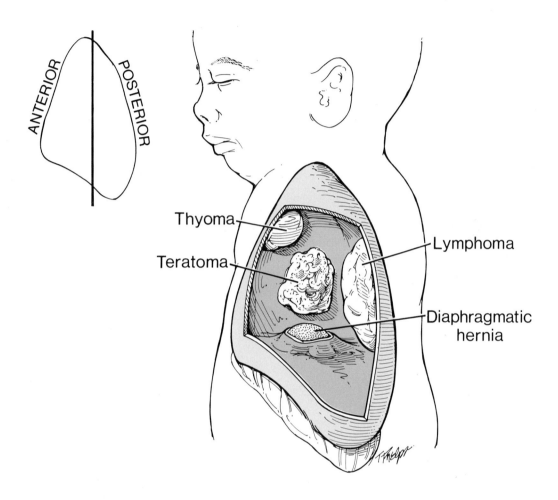

Schematic drawing of the chest and some tumors that may occur in children. The anterior and posterior mediastinal areas are defined in the insets.

chapter **10**

PULMONARY VEINS

The pulmonary veins carry oxygenated blood from the lungs to the morphologic left atrium and from there to the left ventricle and the body. Normally there are four major veins connecting to the left atrium (right and left, upper and lower lobe branches). Pulmonary venous drainage and connection are not synonymous because veins such as the right upper vein may connect normally but, in the presence of an atrial septal defect, they may drain directly into the right atrium.

Pulmonary veins are extracardiac structures but pass through the pericardium connecting to the left atrium. During embryogenesis, the pulmonary veins are incorporated into the back of the morphologic left atrium, so that the back wall of the left atrium is nonmuscular between the entry of the right and left pulmonary vein branches. In congenital anomalies of pulmonary veins with situs solitus of the atria, it is usual for the veins to form a pulmonary-venous confluence first and then connect abnormally. When there is atrial situs ambiguous (right or left atrial isomerism), the pulmonary venous connection is more variable (see further on).

The tomographic planes used to image the pulmonary veins and their connections are variations of coronal planes. A plane passing through the connections of all four veins is nearly vertical and in most patients can be obtained by ultrasonography by positioning from the suprasternal notch.[1-4] In practice the right and left veins are visualized better individually (Plates XXII and XXIII).

NORMAL MORPHOLOGY AND CONNECTIONS

The four pulmonary veins return symmetrically to the left atrium, which is located in the heart of the chest. There is variability in the orientation of the pulmonary veins as they travel to the left atrium, but the upper lobe veins are oriented in a plane ranging from 0 to 45 degrees from a transverse plane (Figure 10–1). Normally there are four major veins, but there may be an accessory vein from the right middle lobe that can be identified in ultrasound scans. The right and left pulmonary veins can enter as a single vein. The ultrasonic appearance of successive scans of the normal right and left pulmonary veins is shown in Figure 10–2.

RIGHT UPPER PULMONARY VEIN

The right upper pulmonary vein enters the right, superior aspect of the left atrium. This entry can be seen reliably from both the subcostal and suprasternal approaches. From the latter approach both the upper and lower veins on the right can be seen in the same scan, so there is less chance of confusion between the two than in other scans. In suprasternal scans the right upper vein is posterior to the right pulmonary artery, and this relationship holds for the other veins as well. The right pulmonary artery, therefore, serves as a reliable marker in the chest during suprasternal scanning. By tilting the transducer slightly posterior to it, one can visualize the most posterior aspect of the left atrium and the right pulmonary veins connecting to it. The angle of entry into the left atrium is 30

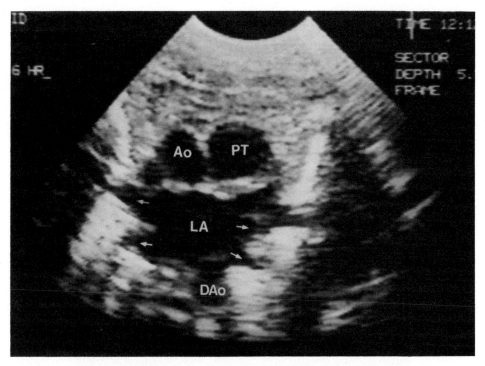

FIG. 10–1. High parasternal scans of the pulmonary veins entering the left atrium (LA). Note the entry angle of the veins and the possibility of confusion between the site of entry of the left upper pulmonary vein and the left atrial appendage.

to 45 degrees and makes this vein poorly suited for routine Doppler sampling of pulmonary venous flow velocity from a suprasternal approach, but it can be done in cooperative infants and children. The subcostal or apical position allows placement of a pulsed Doppler sample volume near the site of entry of the right upper vein (Figure 10–3).

Partial anomalous connection of this vein is almost always to the right superior vena cava and is frequently associated with an atrial septal defect of the sinus venosus type.

RIGHT LOWER PULMONARY VEIN

The right lower pulmonary vein drains about two thirds of the right lung and is normally slightly larger than the upper vein. It enters the left atrium at its right lower corner, usually at an angle of 20 to 30 degrees to the horizontal plane. Because of anatomic factors, it is relatively easy to image this vein from the suprasternal approach and to obtain a Doppler velocity tracing in it.

Partial anomalous connection of this vein is most often directly to the right atrium or the inferior vena cava at its junction with the right atrium. One clue to this problem is the contour of the back of the left atrium that results from normal "tethering" of each of its corners. Lack of normal entry of a vein will result in loss of one the "corners" of the left atrium (see below).

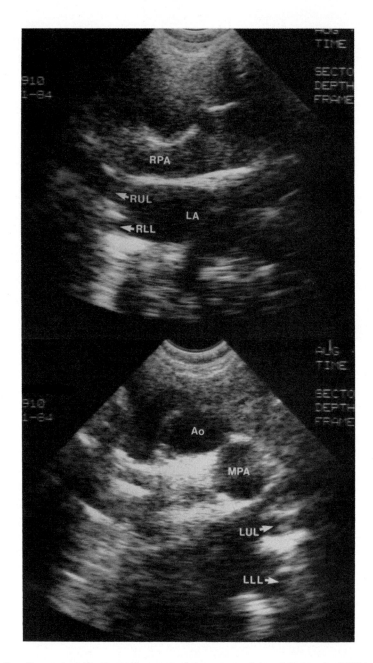

FIG. 10–2. Suprasternal ultrasonic scan of the entry of the right upper (RUL) and right lower (RLL) pulmonary veins into the left atrium (LA) (upper panel). With slight counterclockwise rotation of the transducer, the left upper (LUL) and left lower (LLL) pulmonary veins can also be imaged behind the main pulmonary artery (MPA) (lower panel).

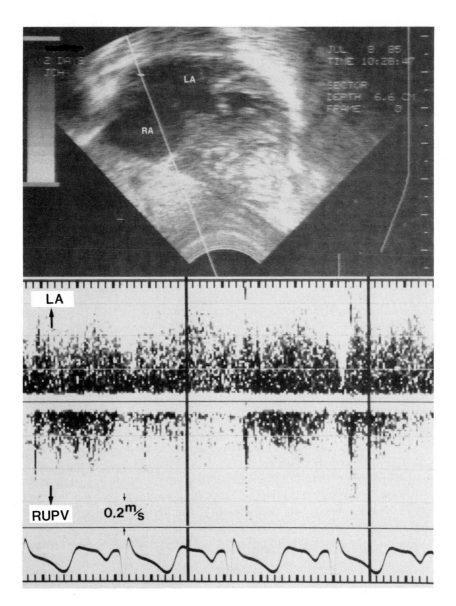

FIG. 10–3. Apical scanning of the left and right atria with the pulsed Doppler sample volume placed in the right upper pulmonary vein (upper panel). The blood flow velocity pattern oriented toward the transducer (lower panel) was nearly continuous in this patient, who had a large left-to-right shunt from a ventricular septal defect.

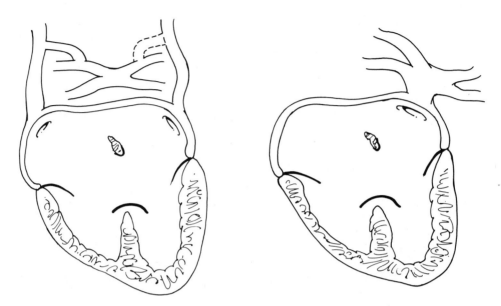

FIG. 10–4. Pulmonary venous connection pattern found in patients with right atrial iso-merism. The pulmonary veins connect to a pulmonary venous confluence, which then drains to either of the superior cavae (left) or to either of the morphologic right atria (right).

LEFT UPPER PULMONARY VEIN

This vein enters the left atrium immediately behind the left atrial appendage in the left posterior and superior corner. During ultrasound examination of the pulmonary veins, it is common to mistake the orifice of the left atrial appendage for the left upper pulmonary vein. Therefore it is important to image both structures simultaneously. Isolated stenosis of this vein may be difficult to di-agnose by ultrasound without Doppler assistance because its orifice may appear narrow only in some views; however, Doppler assessment should be useful in this regard. Partial anomalous connection of the left upper pulmonary vein is almost always to the more superior left innominate vein. This accompanies the most common type of mixed total anomalous pulmonary venous connection.

LEFT LOWER PULMONARY VEIN

The left lower pulmonary vein normally connects to the left posteroinferior aspect of the left atrium. The course of this vein is anterior to the descending aorta and posterior to the left pulmonary artery. This pulmonary vein may enter the left atrium, forming an infolding of pericardial reflection, which can simulate cor triatriatum (two left atrial chambers). Rarely, such an atrial wall infolding can cause cor triatriatum, but it is unlike the classic form in which a membrane causes the obstruction.

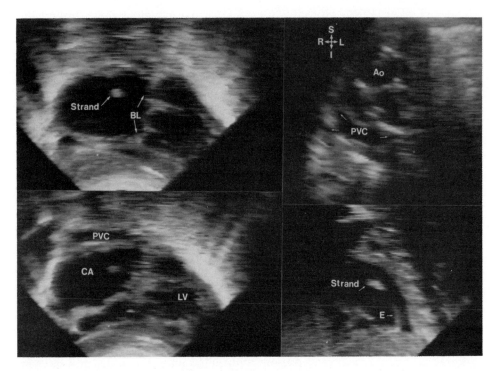

FIG. 10–5. Abnormal pulmonary venous connection in a patient with asplenia syndrome and a common atrioventricular valve. Bilateral right atria are suspected because of the presence of an atrial strand (left upper panel), and a pulmonary venous confluence (PVC) without obvious connection to either atrium is imaged from subcostal (left lower panel) and suprasternal (right upper panel) scans. The atrial strand appeared to be related to the eustachian valve (E) (right lower panel). CA = common atrium; BL = bridging leaflet. (From Br Heart J 53:525, 1985.)

Partial anomalous connection of this vein is rare and is usually to the coronary sinus.

ANOMALOUS PULMONARY VENOUS CONNECTION

Anomalous pulmonary venous connection is classified into partial and total. With total anomalous pulmonary venous connection all four pulmonary veins connect to a structure other than the morphologic left atrium. Such patients present in infancy with congestive heart failure or cyanosis or both and frequently need emergency surgery. Partial anomalous pulmonary venous connection means that at least one pulmonary vein connects abnormally while at least one vein connects to the morphologic left atrium. Such patients may be asymptomatic and the condition may only be recognized because of coexisting congenital heart disease. Isolated partial anomalous pulmonary venous connection is rarely diagnosed[5] and is usually diagnosed at autopsy.

Definition of anomalous pulmonary venous connection becomes difficult in the case of atrial-visceral situs ambiguous[6] (which is actually not ambiguous but is either right or left atrial isomerism). When there are two right atria and no morphologic left atrium there is, by the above definition, total anomalous pulmonary venous connection. This is true even though the pulmonary venous *drainage* is to the left-sided atrium. Careful pathologic and ultrasonic examination of the patterns of connection in right atrial isomerism (also called asplenia syndrome) shows that the veins enter a confluence before entry into one of the cavae or either of the morphologic right atria (Figure 10–4). Bilateral right atria can be recognized by the appearance of the atrial appendages (see Chapter 11) or by the presence of an atrial strand in what appears to be a common atrium (Figure 10–5).

Likewise, with bilateral left atria (sometimes referred to as polysplenia syndrome) the pulmonary veins may connect to the left-sided morphologic left atrium or to both atria.

PARTIAL ANOMALOUS CONNECTION

Diagnosis of *partial anomalous venous connection* has been attempted using digital subtraction angiography.[7] Ultrasonic contrast techniques during cardiac catheterization may be the most accurate way of defining the exact site of connection of an anomalous pulmonary vein.[8]

Partial anomalous pulmonary venous connection can occur with sequestration in the lung. Such infants may present with pulmonary difficulties and have an abnormal arterial supply of a portion of lung from the descending aorta and pulmonary venous connection from it to the right atrium. A well-recognized form of this abnormality is *scimitar syndrome*. On chest radiographs the anomalous pulmonary veins on the right form a curvilinear density paralleling the right atrial shadow that resembles a scimitar.[9] This diagnosis is usually suspected on the chest x-ray, and cross-sectional imaging may be useful to diagnose the number of pulmonary veins connecting normally.

Anomalous connection of only the *right upper pulmonary vein* to the right superior vena cava may be a common lesion that has little significance because it has been recognized as an incidental finding in autopsy studies of normal adults who have died in accidents. This anomalous connection usually occurs with sinus venosus atrial septal defect. Sinus venosus atrial septal defect produces characteristic ultrasonic features but may be difficult to diagnose if imaging is of poor quality.[10] Using suprasternal scans, the right superior vena caval–right atrial junction and the anomalous connection behind the right pulmonary artery can be imaged.

Partial anomalous connections of the *left pulmonary veins* are almost entirely to the left innominate vein and to the coronary sinus with or without a persistent left superior vena cava. In sequestration of the left lower lobe of the lung, the signs of absence of normal left lower vein connection may be present (Figure 10–6).

TOTAL ANOMALOUS CONNECTION

The aim of ultrasound imaging in *total anomalous pulmonary venous connection* is to confirm the diagnosis, which often is suspected clinically in a neonate or

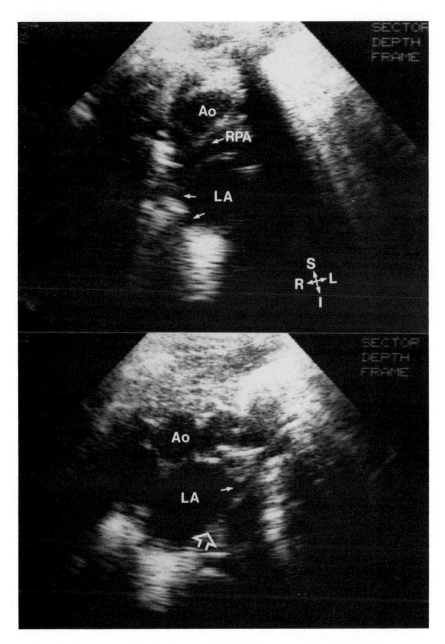

FIG. 10–6. Absence of normal pulmonary venous connection of the left lower pulmonary vein in a patient with sequestration of the left lower lobe of the left lung. Suprasternal scans revealed normal right pulmonary venous connection (upper panel); however, scans of the left-sided pulmonary veins revealed normal connection of only the left upper pulmonary vein (small white arrow in the lower panel). The site of expected left lower pulmonary venous connection is shown with the open white arrow.

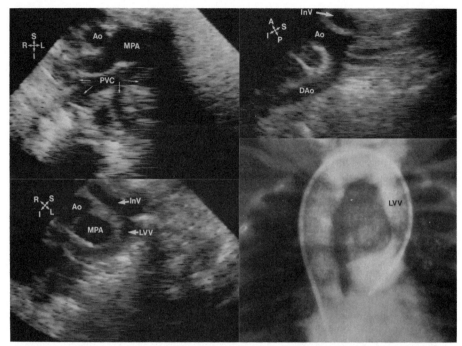

FIG. 10–7. Total anomalous pulmonary venous connection to a left vertical vein in an infant. Suprasternal scans reveal the entry of the four pulmonary veins to the pulmonary venous confluence (PVC) (left upper panel), and segmental imaging of the vertical vein and innominate vein (InV) confirm the diagnosis. An angiogram with the catheter in the left vertical vein (LVV) is shown for comparison (right lower panel). (From Br Heart J *53*:525, 1985.)

infant with congestive heart failure and cardiomegaly. In addition, all four pulmonary veins should be imaged and their connections defined. When this cannot be achieved with confidence, then angiography is necessary to exclude unusual anomalies such as variations of the mixed type of total anomalous pulmonary venous connection. Over a 29-month period at Texas Children's Hospital, a study of the diagnosis of total anomalous pulmonary venous connection revealed that cross-sectional ultrasound imaging was highly accurate except in three circumstances: (1) abnormal atrial situs, (2) complex congenital heart disease with pulmonary atresia, and (3) pulmonary vein atresia.[11]

Total anomalous pulmonary venous connection with situs solitus of the atria is classified into four subgroups: (1) supracardiac, (2) intracardiac, (3) infracardiac, and (4) mixed. Common features of total anomalous pulmonary venous connection on ultrasound imaging of the heart shared by many types include right ventricular enlargement with compression of the left ventricle, making it appear relatively hypoplastic; right atrial enlargement with deviation of the interatrial septum to the left; and enlargement of the pulmonary arteries. However, confident diagnosis depends on direct visualization of the pulmonary veins and their connections.[12,13] Confirmatory Doppler ultrasound features include a pattern of main pulmonary flow velocity suggestive of large flow and pulmonary hypertension and identification of increased flow velocity at the site of pulmonary venous connection.

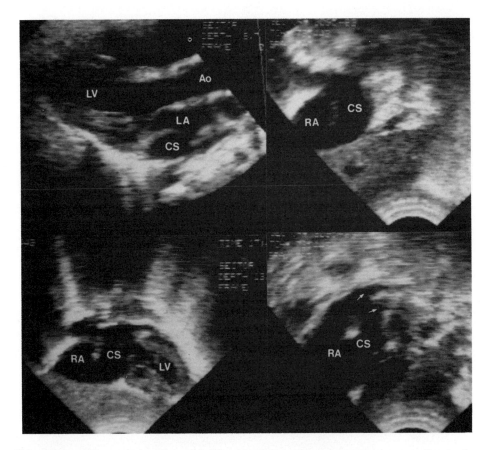

FIG. 10–8.   Ultrasonic imaging of total anomalous pulmonary venous connection to the coronary sinus. Long axis scans show a markedly dilated coronary sinus behind the left atrium (left upper panel). Imaging of the entry of the pulmonary veins into the coronary sinus (white arrows) is possible from subcostal scans. (From Br Heart J 53:525, 1985.)

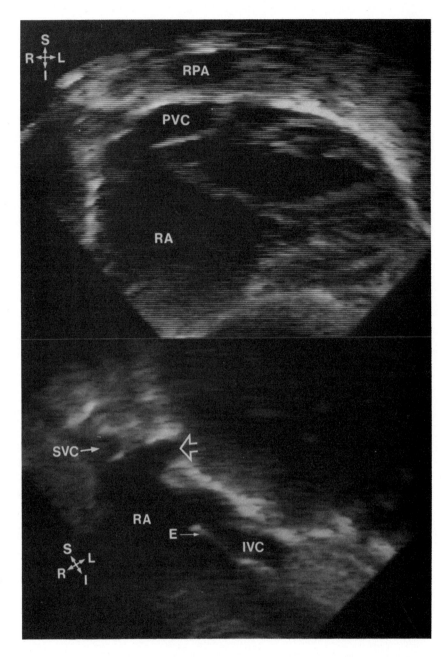

FIG. 10–9. Ultrasonic imaging of total anomalous pulmonary venous connection to the right atrium. Subcostal scans reveal the pulmonary venous confluence (PVC) connecting to the junction of the right atrium (PA) with the right superior vena cava (upper panel). This is confirmed in a sagittal subcostal scan, with the inferior vena cava (IVC), superior vena cava (SVC), and eustachian valve simultaneously imaged (lower panel). (From Br Heart J *53*:525, 1985.)

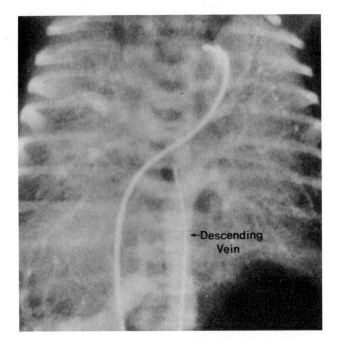

FIG. 10–10. Angiographic findings in a patient with total anomalous pulmonary venous connection below the diaphragm via a descending vein, following a pulmonary angiogram.

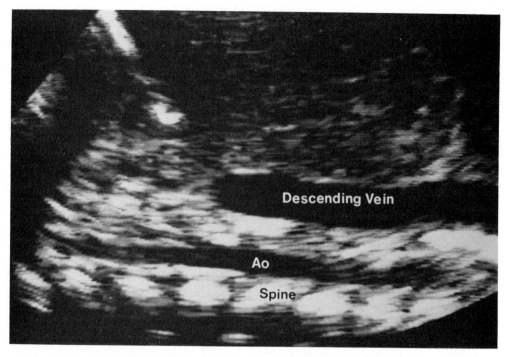

FIG. 10–11. Sagittal scan of the abdomen showing the descending aorta, spine, and more anterior descending vein entering the liver.

Supracardiac total anomalous pulmonary venous connection is to one of the systemic veins above the diaphragm (see Chapter 11). The most common site of supracardiac connection is the *left vertical vein* with subsequent drainage to the innominate vein, the right superior vena cava, and then the right atrium. Such a pulmonary venous confluence can be visualized by cross-sectional imaging from the subcostal or suprasternal approach using coronal scans. However, mapping the course of the subsequent drainage requires multiple projections (Figure 10–7). Doppler ultrasound has been shown to be useful in such patients by diagnosing the direction of blood flow in the left vertical vein as superior rather than inferior, as in the left superior vena cava to the coronary sinus.[14] Other less common sites of supracardiac connection of a pulmonary venous confluence such as the *right superior vena cava* or the *azygos vein* are frequently associated with narrowing at the site of entry. In cases of pulmonary venous obstruction, careful scanning of the confluence and the course of the connection can direct the use of Doppler sampling in search of a high velocity jet.

Intracardiac total anomalous venous connection is most likely to the *coronary sinus*, and in such cases subcostal scanning planes are especially useful. A dilated coronary sinus may be attributable to many causes, so it is important to directly image the pulmonary veins connecting to the coronary sinus (Figure 10–8). When all four pulmonary veins connect to the coronary sinus there rarely is pulmonary venous obstruction, and such infants present with failure to thrive

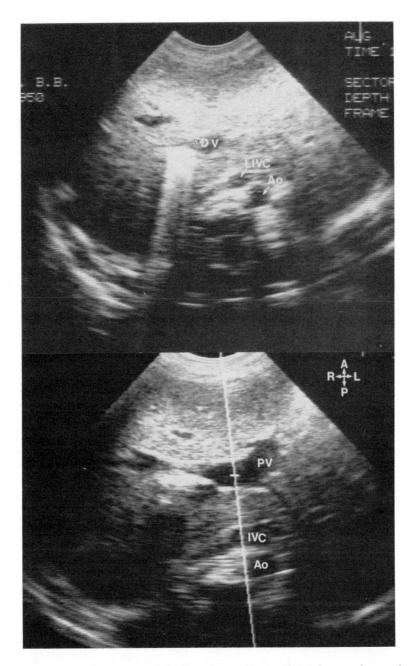

FIG. 10–12. Transverse scans of the liver in a patient with total anomalous pulmonary venous connection below the diaphragm. The descending vein (DV) is anterior to the aorta and inferior vena cava and connects to a dilated portal vein (PV) (lower panel). This patient had right atrial isomerism, with the left-sided inferior vena cava (LIVC) and aorta (Ao) running together.

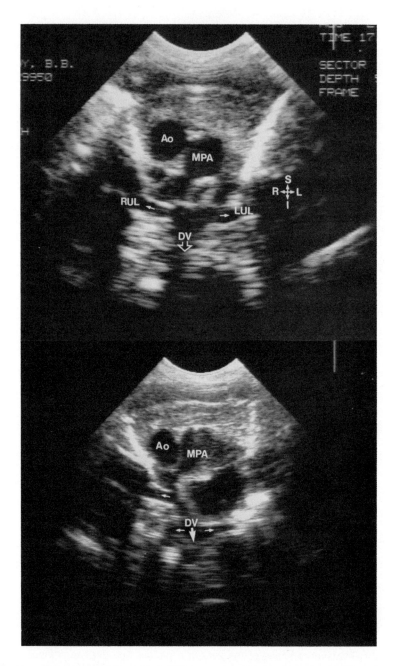

FIG. 10–13.   Suprasternal imaging of total anomalous pulmonary venous connection showing the connection of the right upper and left upper pulmonary veins to the descending vein (upper panel). The lower lobe pulmonary venous connection can be imaged with more posterior orientation of the transducer (small white arrows in the lower panel).

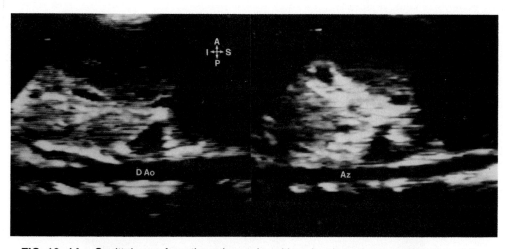

FIG. 10–14. Sagittal scan from the subcostal position showing azygos continuation of the inferior vena cava (Az), which should not be confused with the descending vein in total anomalous pulmonary venous connection. Note the more posterior position of the azygos continuation compared with the nearby descending aorta (DAo) (left panel).

syndrome and congestive heart failure. The other common site of anomalous pulmonary venous connection is the *right atrium.* In this type the pulmonary veins most often connect to a confluence and then drain to the right atrium (Figure 10–9).

Infracardiac total anomalous pulmonary venous connection is uncommon and almost always obstructed. Consequently, the patient with this entity presents in the neonatal period with severe cyanosis and lack of cardiac dilation, which may simulate pulmonary disease.[15] The most common site of connection in this group is the *portal vein* in the liver. This connection can be diagnosed by ultrasonography using subcostal transverse and sagittal scans to image the vein descending to the liver through the diaphragm (Figures 10–10 and 10–11). This is straightforward because the descending vein is anterior to the aorta and inferior vena cava on transverse scans (Figure 10–12).[16] All four pulmonary veins must be imaged connecting to the confluence, which is best seen on suprasternal scans (Figure 10–13). It is important to distinguish this descending vein from other anomalous veins traversing the diaphragm, such as azygos continuation of the inferior vena cava (Figure 10–14). Doppler may be useful in assessing the blood flow velocity in the descending vein (Figure 10–15). Other less common sites of connection are the *inferior vena cava,* a *hepatic vein,* or the *ductus venosus.*

Mixed total anomalous pulmonary venous connection made up 6% of all forms of total anomalous connection in our recent series[11] and the most common type was to the *left vertical vein and the coronary sinus.* This anomaly is made more complex by variations in the interconnection of the left and right pulmonary veins (Figures 10–16 and 10–17).

STENOSIS

Pulmonary vein stenosis can be diagnosed by Doppler techniques, and in a recent review of our experience we noted that a continuous wave velocity greater

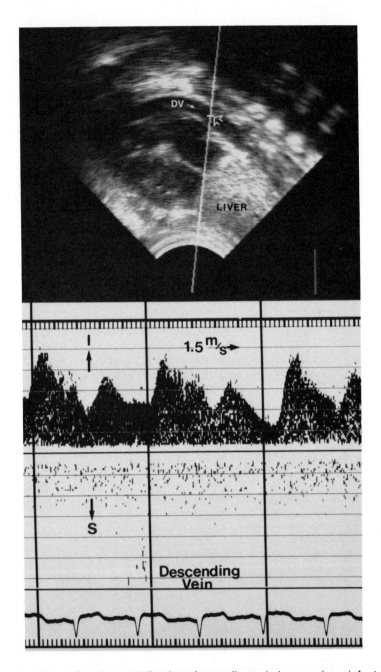

FIG. 10–15. Pulsed Doppler sampling in a descending vein in a newborn infant with total anomalous pulmonary venous connection below the diaphragm. Note the inferiorly oriented blood flow with a peak velocity of 1.5 m/sec.

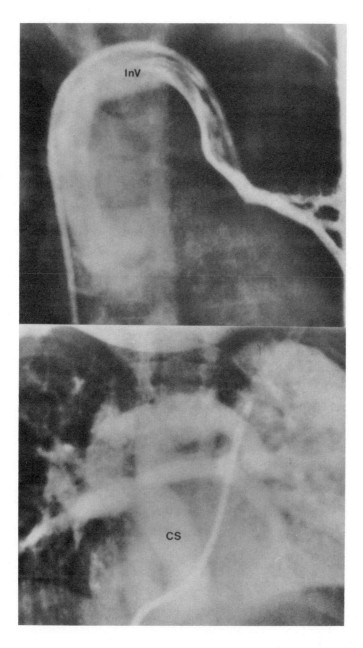

FIG. 10–16. Angiographic findings in a patient with total anomalous pulmonary venous connection of the mixed type. Note the left lung veins connecting to a left vertical vein and innominate vein (InV) (upper panel) and the right-sided pulmonary veins and lower pulmonary veins connecting to the coronary sinus (CS) (lower panel). (From Br Heart J 53:525, 1985.)

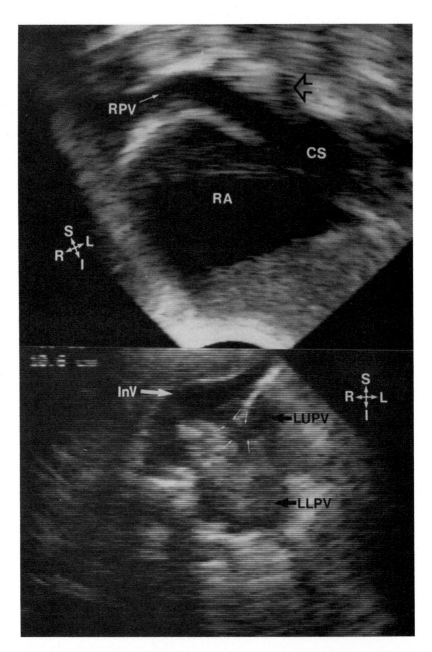

FIG. 10–17. Corresponding ultrasonic scans in a patient with mixed total anomalous pulmonary venous connection. The right pulmonary venous connection to the coronary sinus and the left lower pulmonary venous connection (open black arrow) are imaged (upper panel). The left upper pulmonary venous connection to the innominate vein (InV) is also seen (lower panel). (From Br Heart J *53*:525, 1985.)

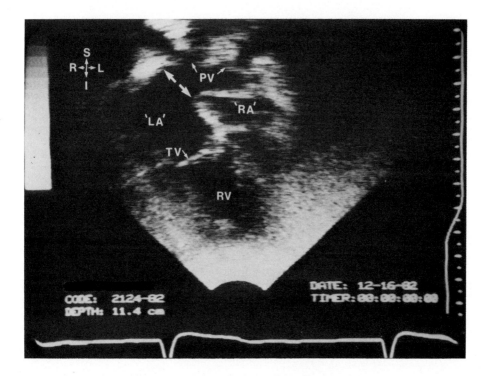

FIG. 10–18.   Apical imaging of a patient following the Mustard procedure for transposition of the great arteries. The new pulmonary venous pathway (white arrows) is widely patent, and the return of the pulmonary veins to the new left atrium (LA) is unobstructed.

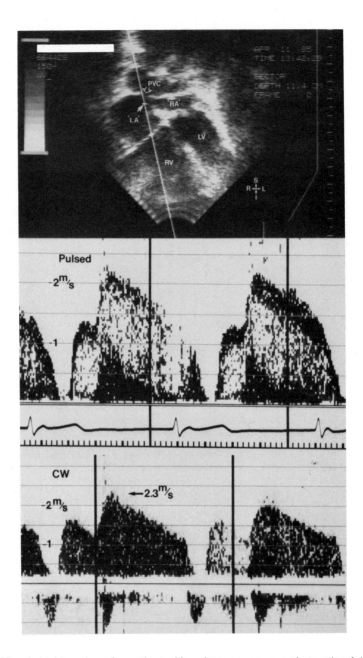

FIG. 10–19. Apical imaging of a patient with pulmonary venous obstruction following the Mustard procedure. The narrow orifice between the pulmonary venous confluence and the new left atrium (open white arrow) can be imaged (upper panel). Pulsed Doppler (middle panel) and continuous wave Doppler (lower panel) sampling at this site show increased velocity compatible with severe pulmonary venous obstruction.

than 2.0 m/sec reliably predicted a gradient of at least 16 mm Hg across the stenosis. Pulsed Doppler sampling in the orifice of the entry of the vein into the left atrium shows an increased, continuous velocity.

Following an intra-atrial transposition of venous return (Mustard or Senning operation) for transposition of the great arteries, pulmonary venous obstruction may result. Ultrasonic imaging of the region of the posterior pathway of pulmonary venous return to the new left atrium (LA) and the tricuspid valve can exclude this diagnosis when a widely patent pathway can be seen (Figure 10–18). When this is not the case, Doppler sampling using pulsed and continuous-wave techniques can make the diagnosis of obstruction (Figure 10–19).

ATRESIA

Pulmonary vein atresia may affect all the veins and lead to rapid death shortly after birth.[17] Ultrasonic imaging can be used when this diagnosis is suspected.[11] However, it would be difficult to find a survivor of cardiac surgery for this condition. The venous return is usually via bronchial veins.

Atresia of the left or right pulmonary veins results in hypoplasia of the ipsilateral pulmonary artery, which may be a clue to the diagnosis using noninvasive techniques.

REFERENCES

 1. Goldberg BB: Suprasternal ultrasonography. JAMA 215:245, 1971.
 2. Allen HD, Goldberg SJ, Sahn DJ, et al: Suprasternal notch echocardiography: Assessment of its clinical utility in pediatric cardiology. Circulation 55:605, 1977.
 3. Goh TH, and Venables AW: Scanning suprasternal echocardiography. Br Heart J 43:95, 1980.
 4. Snider AR, and Silverman NH: Suprasternal notch echocardiography: A two-dimensional technique for evaluating congenital heart disease. Circulation 63:165, 1981.
 5. Stewart JR, Schaff HV, Fortuin, NJ, and Brawley RK: Partial anomalous pulmonary venous return with intact atrial septum: Report of four cases. Thorax 38:859, 1983.
 6. Macartney FJ, Zuberbuhler JR, and Anderson RH: Morphological considerations pertaining to recognition of atrial isomerism. Consequences for sequential chamber localisation. Br Heart J 44:657, 1980.
 7. Snider AR, Enderlein MA, Teitel DF, and Juster RP: Two-dimensional echocardiographic determination of aortic and pulmonary artery sizes from infancy to adulthood in normal subjects. Am J Cardiol 53:218, 1984.
 8. Danilowicz D, and Kronzon I: Use of contrast echocardiography in the diagnosis of partial anomalous pulmonary venous connection. Am J Cardiol 43:248, 1979.
 9. Stocker JT, and Malczak HT: A study of pulmonary ligament arteries. Relationship to intralobar pulmonary sequestration. Chest 86:611, 1984.
10. Nasser FN, Tajik AJ, Seward JB, and Hagler DJ: Diagnosis of sinus venosus atrial septal defect by two-dimensional echocardiography. Mayo Clin Proc 56:568, 1981.
11. Huhta JC, Gutgesell HP, and Nihill MR: Cross-sectional echocardiographic diagnosis of total anomalous pulmonary venous connection. Br Heart J 53:525, 1985.
12. Sahn DJ, Allen HD, McDonald G, and Goldberg SJ: Real-time cross-sectional echocardiographic diagnosis of the site of total anomalous pulmonary venous drainage (TAPVD). Circulation 60:1317, 1979.
13. Smallhorn JF, Sutherland GR, Tommasini G, et al: Assessment of total anomalous pulmonary venous connection by two-dimensional echocardiography. Br Heart J 46:613, 1981.
14. Skovranek J, Tuma S, Urbancova D, and Samanek M: Range-gated pulsed Doppler echocardiographic diagnosis of supracardiac total anomalous pulmonary venous drainage. Circulation 61:841, 1980.

15. Long WA, Lawson EE, Harned HS Jr, and Henry GW: Infradiaphragmatic total anomalous pulmonary venous drainage: New diagnostic, physiologic, and surgical considerations. Am J Perinatol 1:227, 1984.
16. Huhta JC, Smallhorn JF, and Macartney FJ: Cross-sectional echocardiographic diagnosis of azygos continuation of the inferior vena cava. Cathet Cardiovasc Diagn 10:221, 1984.
17. Khonsari S, Saunders PW, Lees MH, and Starr A: Common pulmonary vein atresia. Importance of immediate recognition and surgical intervention. J Thorac Cardiovasc Surg 83:443, 1982.

chapter **11**

SYSTEMIC VEINS

Abnormalities of systemic venous return to the heart are common and occur with, and without, congenital heart disease. Accurate diagnosis of these entities is important in children for several reasons: (1) the appearance of some abnormalities on ultrasound imaging may be incorrectly diagnosed as serious cardiac or pulmonary disease, (2) venous abnormalities may affect the management of children with congenital heart disease during cardiac catheterization, and (3) failure to identify a venous structure or abnormal connection may adversely affect cardiac surgery or other procedures such as permanent pacemaker implantation.

NORMAL VENOUS RETURN

Normal systemic venous connection may be defined *segmentally* for patients with atrial situs solitus as right superior vena caval connection to the right atrium with a left innominate vein but no left superior vena cava, coronary sinus connection to the right atrium, inferior vena caval connection to the right atrium, and hepatic venous connection to the inferior vena cava. Many ultrasound scanning planes are needed to make this determination but, with experience, it can be accomplished in one or two minutes.

Diagnosis of systemic venous return should be done according to a systematic, segmental method. Each normal structure should be imaged routinely during every examination. The diagnostic method for systemic venous return requires investigation of: (1) the presence or absence of each venous segment, and (2) the connection of each. Tomographic planes that can be used to image these venous segments are illustrated in Plates XXIV, XXV, and XXVI.

SITUS DIAGNOSIS

Normal systemic venous return cannot be identified without knowledge of the atrial situs. For example, a pattern of venous connection that may be abnormal in atrial situs solitus may be entirely appropriate for right atrial isomerism.[1] The common patterns of venous return in abnormal atrial situs are shown in Figure 11–1.

In situs that is normal (situs solitus) the inferior vena cava ascends on the right, receives hepatic venous connection, and enters the right atrium. The eustachian valve is a helpful marker of this entry and of the morphologic right atrium.[2] In situs inversus totalis the inferior vena cava ascends on the patient's left side and the atria and thorax are a mirror image of normal. Situs solitus and inversus are examples of lateralized situs. This lateralization extends to the lungs (bi-lobed on the left and tri-lobed on the right in situs solitus) and the bronchi (hyparterial on the left and eparterial on the right).

In right atrial isomerism there is usually asplenia, bilateral eparterial bronchi, and complex congenital heart disease. The inferior vena cava may be left- or right-sided, connects with some hepatic veins, and enters the midportion of a common atrium. This last term is a misnomer, since there usually is an atrial strand of muscle instead of a normal atrial septum separating the two morpho-

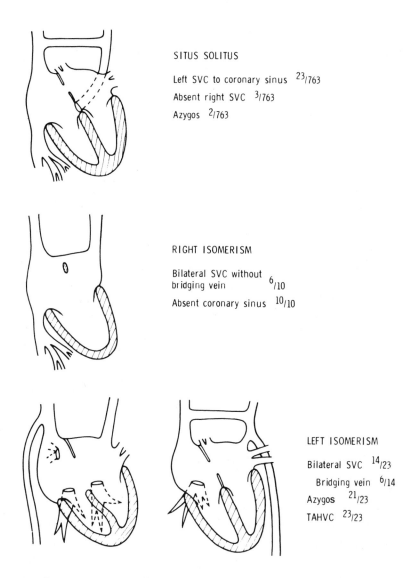

SITUS SOLITUS

Left SVC to coronary sinus   23/763

Absent right SVC   3/763

Azygos   2/763

RIGHT ISOMERISM

Bilateral SVC without
bridging vein   6/10

Absent coronary sinus   10/10

LEFT ISOMERISM

Bilateral SVC   14/23

Bridging vein   6/14

Azygos   21/23

TAHVC   23/23

FIG. 11–1.   Common patterns of venous return in normal and abnormal atrial situs. (From Br Heart J *48*:388, 1982.)

logic right atria (Figure 11–2). We have also observed that there may be two eustachian valves, one on either side of the entry site of the inferior vena cava.

The position of the aorta, with respect to the inferior vena cava, is highly suggestive of right atrial isomerism. The inferior cava and aorta run together to the left or right of the spine. The inferior vena cava is lateral and anterior to the aorta, presenting a typical appearance on subcostal transverse scans. If the side of the aortic arch is opposite the side of the inferior vena cava, the aorta will "seek out" the cava below the diaphragm, crossing abruptly from one side to the other.[3–5] In left atrial isomerism the inferior vena cava is usually interrupted (see further on), and inferior venous drainage is via an azygos vein (see below).

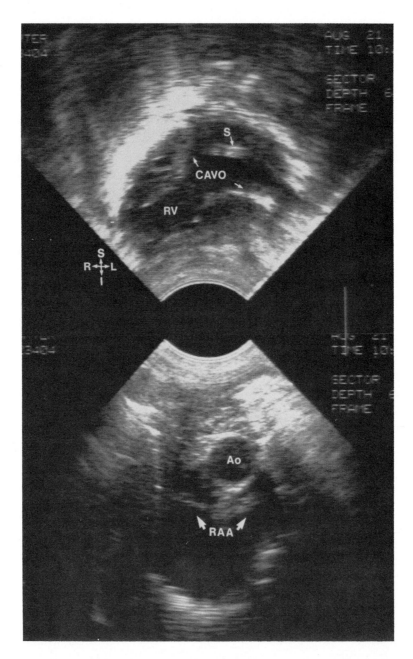

FIG. 11–2. Ultrasonic scanning of the intracardiac anatomy of a patient with right atrial isomerism and an intra-atrial strand in a common atrium (upper panel). The patient has dextrocardia and a common inlet right ventricle. Bilateral right atrial appendages are present (lower panel).

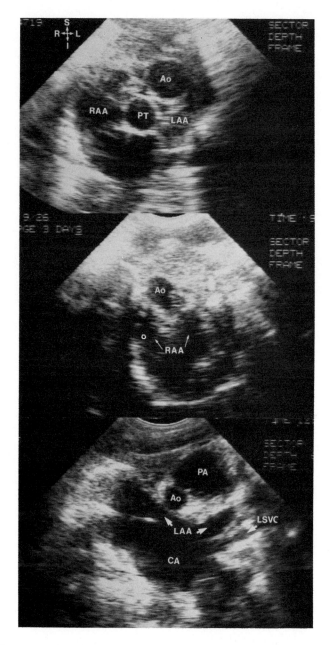

FIG. 11–3. Example of atrial appendage morphology in normal atrial situs (upper panel) and in right (middle panel) and left (lower panel) atrial isomerism. RAA = right atrial appendage; LAA = left atrial appendage.

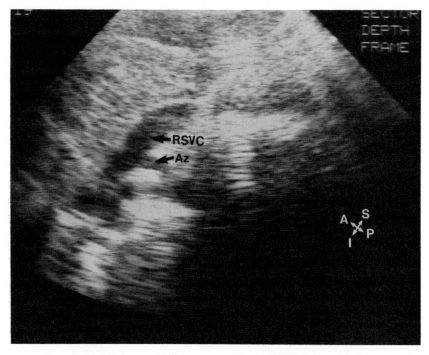

FIG. 11–4. Sagittal scan of the right superior vena cava (RSVC) at the site of normal right azygos vein entry (Az).

This is highly suggestive of bilateral left atria, and the azygos continuation may course on either the left or the right side of the spine.

Direct diagnosis of the atrial situs may be accomplished by visualization of the atrial appendages. This is possible using parasternal, transverse, and sagittal scans (Figure 11–3). The shape of the right atrial appendage resembles a triangle with a broad base, and it has a coarse internal trabecular appearance, while the left atrial appendage has a narrow base and smoother internal features. In atrial isomerism the atrial appendages may not be strictly isomeric, i.e., there may be size differences related to the hemodynamic situation. The shape, internal appearance, and atrial and septal wall morphology will still be diagnostic.

RIGHT SUPERIOR VENA CAVA

The right superior vena cava drains the upper body and connects to the right atrium. It courses in the anterior mediastinum and passes anterior to the right pulmonary artery. It can be imaged from suprasternal scans without difficulty. In coronal scans the right pulmonary artery and aorta serve as useful landmarks when scanning the anterior mediastinum because the right superior cava is to the right of the aorta and anterior to the right pulmonary artery. From sagittal scans the azygos vein, which drains to the right superior vena cava before its entry into the right atrium, can be visualized (Figure 11–4). In this scan the normal right atrial appendage also can be seen and serves as a marker of the morphologic right atrium.

CORONARY SINUS

The coronary sinus receives blood from the coronary veins and returns it to the right atrium. This vein runs in the atrioventricular groove of the heart in a clockwise direction (as viewed from the patient's feet). Congenital or acquired abnormalities of the coronary sinus are rare. Noninvasive imaging of the coronary sinus by cross-sectional ultrasound is straightforward during examination of the heart from the apical and subcostal approaches.[6] The coronary sinus vein is seen entering the right atrium when scanning inferior and posterior to the atrioventricular valves in the plane of the fibrous anuli of the valves and also in parasternal scans (Figure 11–5).

INFERIOR VENA CAVA

Although there are hundreds of variations of normal inferior venous return, there are few significant abnormalities. Ultrasound imaging of the upper portion of the inferior vena cava in children is a routine part of the cardiac and abdominal examinations (Figure 11–6). The inferior venous return has importance for chest examination because the position and connection of this vein are highly useful for the determination of atrial and thoracic situs.

HEPATIC VEINS

The hepatic veins from the left and right lobes of the liver connect normally to the inferior cava. The normal pattern of hepatic venous connection can be imaged from transverse scans of the abdomen near the level of the diaphragm (Figure 11–6).

ABNORMALITIES

LEFT SUPERIOR VENA CAVA

Persistence of the left superior vena cava is the most common type of systemic venous abnormality. It is recognized in association with congenital heart disease in approximately 3% of cases but may occur as an isolated abnormality. In atrial situs solitus a left superior vena cava connects to the coronary sinus and only rarely connects to the left atrium with a normal coronary sinus.

Cross-sectional ultrasound diagnosis of a left superior vena cava is possible using suprasternal and high sagittal scans that show its course anterior to the left pulmonary artery (Figure 11–7).[7] It is important to scan as far to the left as possible to detect a vein that may connect to the innominate vein more toward the left shoulder than usual.

When a left superior vena cava is present, it is necessary to describe the presence or absence of a bridging left innominate vein. This venous segment

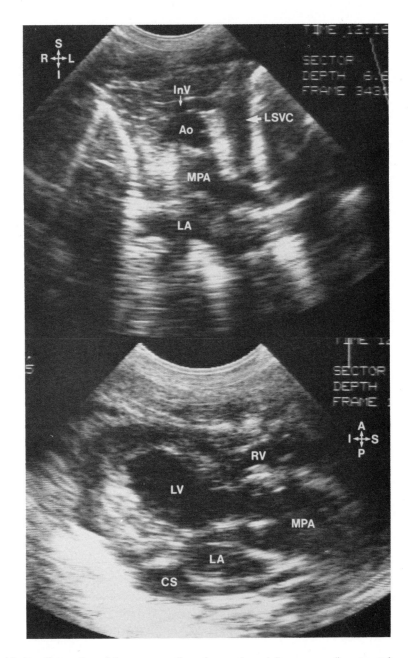

FIG. 11–5. Suprasternal (upper panel) and parasternal (lower panel) scans of a patient with an enlarged left superior vena cava draining to the coronary sinus. The suprasternal scans visualize the innominate vein (InV), the aorta (Ao), the main pulmonary artery (MPA), and the left atrium (LA). The left superior vena cava is well visualized. Imaging of dilation of the coronary sinus and of the left superior vena cava connecting to it behind the left atrium are possible on sagittal scans (lower panel).

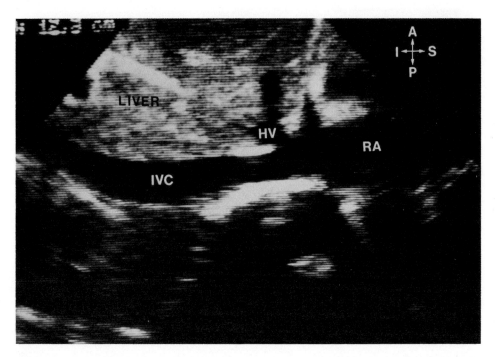

FIG. 11–6. A sagittal scan from the subcostal position showing the inferior vena cava (IVC) connecting to the right atrium (RA). The liver and normal hepatic venous connection (HV) are seen in this scan.

normally connects to the right superior vena cava, so that if there is persistence of the left cava the innominate vein may connect the two venae cavae. Depending on flow patterns, the bridging vein may be quite small or it may be absent. When there is no bridging vein connecting the two cavae, they tend to separate in the upper mediastinum (Figure 11–8), whereas a connecting vein keeps the two veins relatively close together on either side of the aorta. Suprasternal scans are superior in making this determination (Figure 11–9).

Rarely, the innominate vein passes under the aorta rather than over it. Diagnosis of this uncommon entity has usually been made at operation. However, the tomographic modalities such as cross-sectional ultrasound imaging show the position of this structure relative to the aorta in coronal scans (Figure 11–10). Contrast techniques whereby agitated saline is injected into a left arm vein are useful in confirming this rare entity (Figure 11–11).

CORONARY SINUS ABNORMALITIES

The most common abnormality of the *coronary sinus* is enlargement caused by connection to the persistent left superior vena cava. This usually is detected in sagittal or transverse scans of the left ventricle as a circular echolucent structure near the posterior insertion of the mitral valve. Dilation of the coronary sinus also may accompany increased right atrial pressure secondary to right-sided heart failure from any cause. The coronary sinus is absent in many patients with

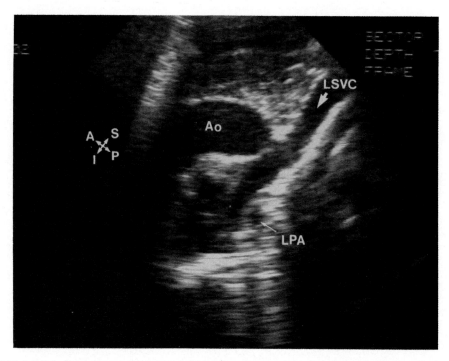

FIG. 11–7. Sagittal scan to the left of the spine showing a left superior vena cava (LSVC) passing anterior to the left pulmonary artery (LPA). A tiny hemiazygos vein is seen connecting to the left superior vena cava immediately above the left pulmonary artery (compare with Figure 11–4).

situs ambiguous, i.e., all of those with right atrial isomerism and over half of those with left atrial isomerism.[1] In the presence of a left superior vena cava this is a strong clue to the abnormal connection of the left cava to the upper portion of the left-side.

A rare but significant congenital abnormality that has not yet been diagnosed noninvasively is atresia of the coronary sinus with coronary venous return to a persistent left superior vena cava.[9] If this abnormality is undetected and the left superior vena cava is ligated during cardiac surgery for other congenital heart disease, there is no exit for obstructed coronary flow, and myocardial function can be seriously compromised.

An uncommon congenital abnormality that causes cyanosis is unroofed coronary sinus with a left superior vena cava.[10] In this anomaly, there is drainage of desaturated left caval blood directly to the left atrium due to a deficiency of tissue between the coronary sinus and the left atrium (Figure 11–12). Scans of the coronary sinus and ultrasound contrast injections in a left arm vein can confirm this diagnosis.

AZYGOS CONTINUATION OF THE INFERIOR VENA CAVA (ABSENCE OF THE HEPATIC SEGMENT OF THE IVC)

This abnormality of venous return is almost always associated with left atrial isomerism. It is significant for the performance of cardiac catheterization in these

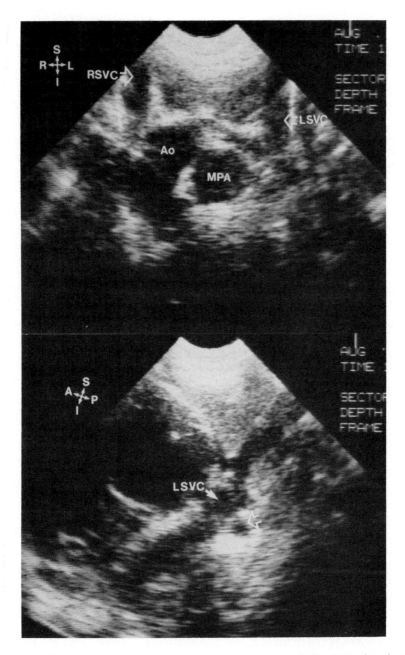

FIG. 11–8. Bilateral superior venae cavae with no bridging vein connecting them. Suprasternal scans (upper panel) make it possible to visualize both structures simultaneously. The course of the left superior vena cava anterior to the left pulmonary artery (open white arrow) is well visualized.

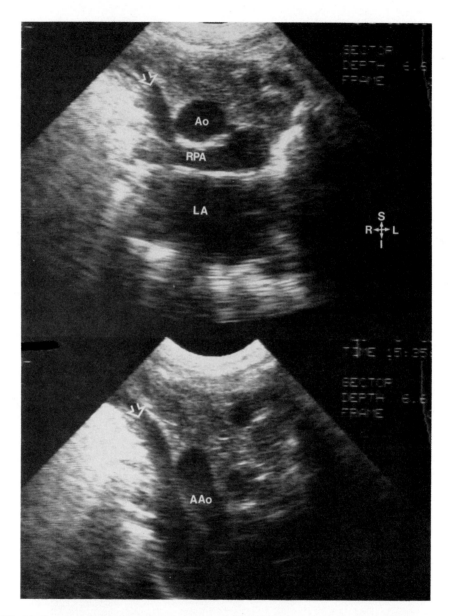

FIG. 11–9. Suprasternal scans of a patient with bilateral superior cavae and no bridging innominate vein. The right superior vena cava (open white arrow) is seen passing anterior to the right pulmonary artery with standard coronal and slightly more anterior scans (lower panel). There is no evidence of an innominate vein.

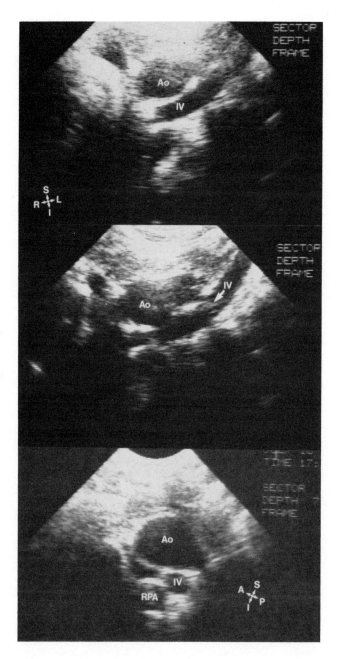

FIG. 11–10. Suprasternal scans of an anomalous course of the innominate vein (IV) under the aortic arch. Coronal sections show the vein passing from the left arm to connect with the right superior vena cava (upper and middle panels). A sagittal scan from the suprasternal approach shows the aorta (Ao) and right pulmonary artery (RPA) in the usual positions, with the innominate vein under the aortic arch adjacent to the right pulmonary artery (lower panel).

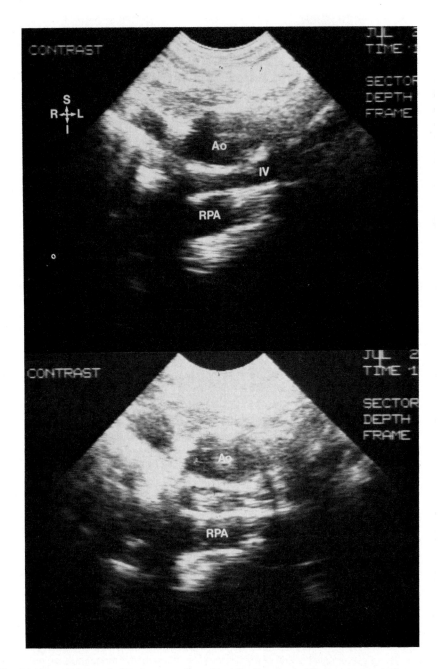

FIG. 11–11. Contrast ultrasonography with injection in a left arm vein during coronal scanning of the anomalous innominate vein described in Figure 11–10. Before (upper panel) and after (lower panel) injection shows opacification of the anomalous vein.

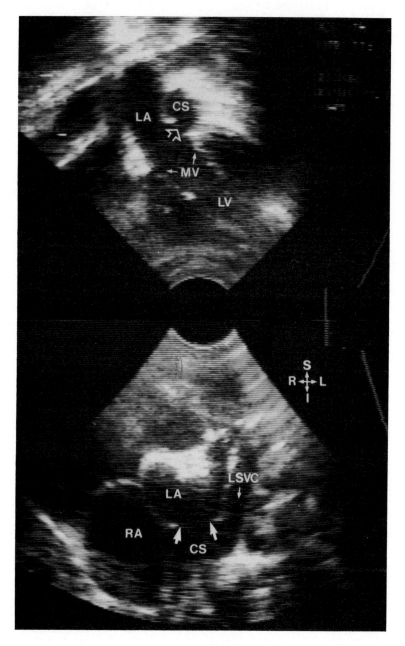

FIG. 11–12. Ultrasound scanning of a patient with unroofed coronary sinus with a left superior vena cava to the coronary sinus. This anomaly allows desaturated left caval blood to drain to the left atrium, causing desaturation. The defect in the roof of the structure is seen in a sagittal scan (lower panel).

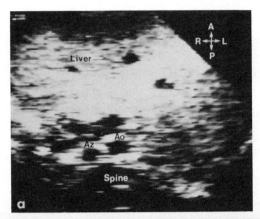

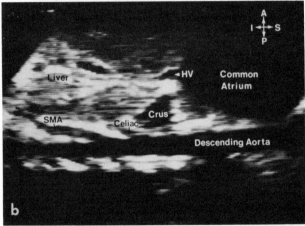

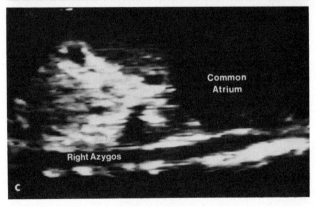

FIG. 11–13. Subcostal imaging of a patient with azygos continuation of the inferior vena cava and abnormal hepatic venous connection to a common atrium. The midline aorta and right posterior position of the azygos vein are well visualized in transverse scans (*a,* upper panel). Scanning of the descending aorta (*b,* middle panel) and the right azygos vein (*c,* lower panel) shows that there is no inferior vena cava connecting to the heart. (From Cathet Cardiovasc Diagn *10:*221, 1984.)

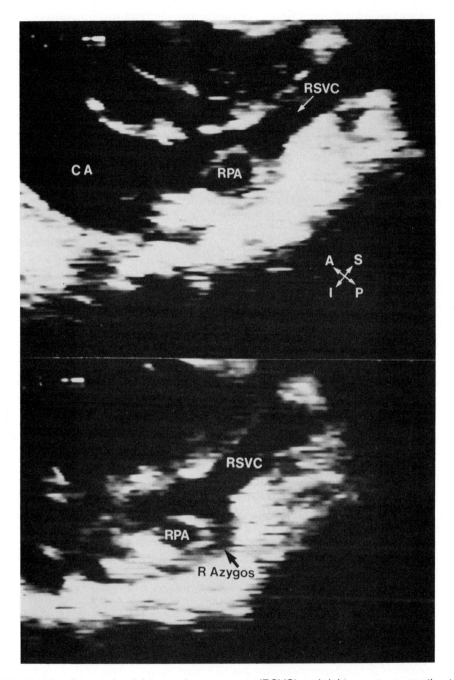

FIG. 11–14. Scans of a right superior vena cava (RSVC) and right azygos connection to it illustrate the right caval connection to a common atrium immediately anterior to the right pulmonary artery (upper panel). The right azygos vein is dilated because of its continuation on the right. (From Cathet Cardiovasc Diagn *10*:221, 1984.)

children because the normal catheter pathway directly to the heart via the inferior vena cava is not available.[11] Special efforts are usually necessary in order to enter the heart in this situation. This posterior structure carries inferior venous blood to the heart by connecting to the ipsilateral superior vena cava and atrium (Figure 11–13). Imaging of this connection is possible from sagittal scans and confirms the presence of an enlarged superior vena cava on the side of the azygos continuation (Figure 11–14). The more posterior structure is the azygos continuation, and the aorta can be identified by its arterial pulsation and the branching of the celiac and superior mesenteric arteries. Associated congenital abnormalities of intracardiac anatomy include atrioventricular septal defect (AV canal) with common atrium, pulmonary stenosis, and congenital complete heart block.

HEPATIC VENOUS ABNORMALITIES

Abnormal connection of the *hepatic veins* is extremely rare in lateralized situs. Partial anomalous hepatic venous connection of one or two hepatic veins directly to the right atrium is uncommon, but does occur in situs solitus and in right atrial isomerism. Total anomalous hepatic venous connection (all the hepatic veins connecting directly to the heart instead of the inferior vena cava) occurs exclusively in left atrial isomerism, with azygos continuation of the inferior cava (Figure 11–15). This connection may be via one or two venous trunks,[1] and these pierce the diaphragm at a site other than is expected for a normal inferior vena cava. During the examination of systemic venous return it is important not to confuse hepatic veins, connecting to the atrium (atria), with pulmonary veins.

DILATION

The right superior vena cava drains the entire upper body. Dilation of this structure usually indicates increased upper body flow, as in an arteriovenous fistula of the head[12] or one of the upper extremities. Dilation may also occur when the systemic venous pressure is markedly elevated or if there is superior vena cava obstruction. Right superior caval size that is smaller than normal indicates decreased flow, as in the case of persistence of the left superior vena cava.

OBSTRUCTION

Following the Mustard operation, for transposition of the great arteries, superior vena caval obstruction may result either early or late. If it occurs immediately after the surgery, the signs of upper body engorgement and cerebral congestion are dramatic. However, if an obstruction develops long after the operation it may be difficult to detect. This problem can be diagnosed using the pulsed-Doppler technique of suprasternal scanning.[13,14] Anomalies of pulmonary venous connection may disturb the Doppler measurements of superior and inferior vena caval flow patterns (see Chapter 10).[15]

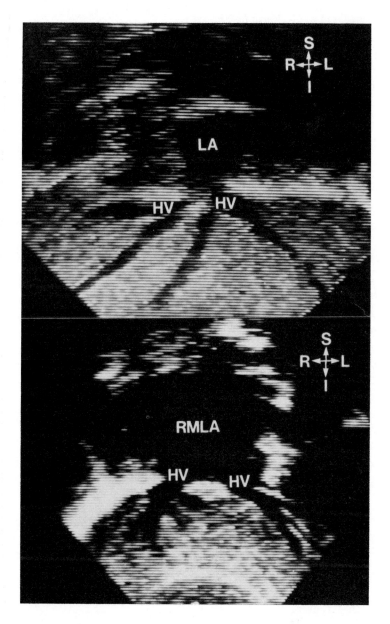

FIG. 11–15. Subcostal scans of anomalous hepatic venous connection with azygos continuation of the inferior vena cava. Symmetrically appearing hepatic right- and left-sided veins connecting to the left-sided left atrium (LA) (upper panel) and right-sided morphologic left atrium (RMLA) (lower panel) are seen. (From Br Heart J *48*:388, 1982.)

REFERENCES

1. Huhta JC, Smallhorn JF, Macartney FJ, et al: Cross-sectional echocardiographic diagnosis of systemic venous return. Br Heart J 48:388, 1982.
2. Limacher MC, Gutgesell HP, Vick GW, et al: Echocardiographic anatomy of the eustachian valve. Am J Cardiol. 57:363, 1986.
3. Elliot LP, Cramer GG, and Amplatz K.: The anomalous relationship of the inferior vena cava and abdominal aorta as a specific angiocardiographic sign in asplenia. Radiology 87:859, 1966.
4. Tonkin IL, and Tonkin AD: Visceroatrial situs abnormalities: Sonographic and computed tomographic appearance. AJR 138:509, 1982.
5. Huhta JC, Smallhorn JF, and Macartney FL: Two-dimensional echocardiographic diagnosis of situs. Br Heart J 48:97, 1982.
6. Snider AR, Ports TA, and Silverman NH: Venous anomalies of the coronary sinus: Detection by M-mode, two-dimensional and contrast echocardiography. Circulation 60:721, 1979.
7. Sanders SP: Echocardiography and related techniques in the diagnosis of congenital heart defects. Part I: Veins, atria and interatrial septum. Echocardiography 1:185, 1984.
8. Smallhorn JF, Zielinsky P, Freedom RM, and Rowe RD: Abnormal position of the brachiocephalic vein. Am J Cardiol 55:234, 1985.
9. Edwards JE: Malformations of the thoracic veins. In Pathology of the Heart, edited by S.E. Gould. 2nd ed., Springfield, Ill., Charles C Thomas, 1960, p. 484.
10. Bourdillon PD, Foale RA, and Somerville J: Persistent left superior vena cava with coronary sinus and left atrial connections. Eur J Cardiol 11:227, 1980.
11. Anderson RC, Adams P Jr, and Burk B: Anomalous inferior vena cava with azygos continuation (infrahepatic interruption of the inferior vena cava). Report of 15 new cases. J Pediatr 59:370, 1961.
12. Snider AR, Solfer SJ, Silverman NH: Detection of intracranial arteriovenous fistula by two-dimensional ultrasonography. Circulation 63:1179, 1981.
13. Stevenson JG, Kawabori I, Guntheroth WG, et al: Pulsed Doppler echocardiographic detection of obstruction of systemic venous return after repair of transposition of the great arteries. Circulation 60:1091, 1979.
14. Wyse RKH, Haworth SG, Taylor JFN, and Macartney FJ: Obstruction of superior vena caval pathway after Mustard's repair: Reliable diagnosis by transcutaneous Doppler ultrasound. Br Heart J 42:162, 1979.
15. Matsuo S, Hayano M, Inoue J, et al: Superior and inferior vena cava flow velocity in patients with anomalous pulmonary vein connection. Jpn Heart J 23:169, 1982.

chapter **12**

PLEURA, PERICARDIUM, AND DIAPHRAGM

The pleuro-pericardial-diaphragm unit forms the fibrous borders of the thorax and delimits the heart, lungs, and abdominal contents. The interfaces between these structures create fibrous planes that reflect ultrasound energy during examination of the chest and may be well visualized under some circumstances. It is important to identify areas of pleural-pericardial ultrasonic reflections that may simulate a thoracic abnormality.

NORMAL

The pleura and pericardium envelop the heart and lungs (Plate XXVII), creating potential spaces and providing a tissue interface for nonirritating independent movement of the heart during emptying and filling and of the lungs during the diaphragmatic movements of breathing. The visceral pleura and pericardium are firmly adherent to the lungs and heart, respectively, and the parietal pleura and pericardium are those structures with free edges in a tomographic section of the chest (Plate XXVIII).

The parietal pleura and pericardium have large numbers of lymphatic channels that drain from the mediastinal and lateral surfaces, and each expiration or increased diastolic filling period forces small amounts of fluid into the lymph system. A negative absorptive pressure in these spaces is maintained by plasma colloid osmotic forces. Increased pressure and fluid in these potential spaces may result from increased capillary pressure, decreased plasma colloid osmotic pressure, increased capillary permeability, or blockage of lymphatics. Normally a small amount of fluid lubricates the pleural and pericardial spaces; however, fluid collection from the above causes, easily detectable by ultrasound, is abnormal (see further on). It is known that the posterior wall of the left ventricle may separate briefly from the pericardium because of the normal amount of lubricating pericardial fluid.[1]

PLEURA

The visceral pleura cover the surface of air-filled lung and normally cannot be imaged by ultrasonography. Normal parietal pleura is extremely thin and near the limits of resolution of ultrasound systems in clinical use. It can be visualized when fluid collections are present on both sides of it, such as where there are combined pericardial and pleural effusions. A pericardial effusion may be simulated by pleural effusion or by ascites.[2,3] When excessive fluid is present, the pleural reflections onto the diaphragm also can be visualized and can create confusion.

Artifactual spaces may be simulated when the pleura is imaged from the suprasternal notch. A lucency that simulates another venous structure is sometimes seen adjacent to the superior vena cava (Figure 12–1).

PERICARDIUM

Normal parietal pericardium reflects from the structures entering the heart, including the great arteries, the systemic veins, and the pulmonary veins. Po-

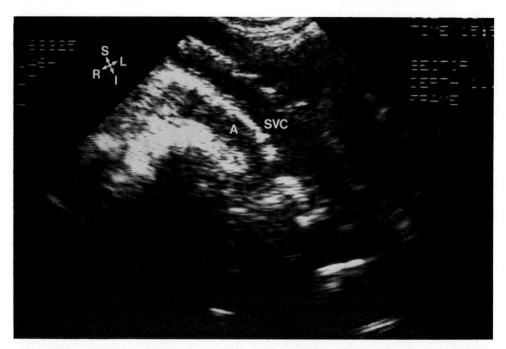

FIG. 12–1. Suprasternal scan showing the right superior vena cava (SVC) and an artifactual echolucent area (A) produced by the junction between the right superior vena cava and the right pleural reflection.

tentially confusing ultrasound imaging findings occur at these sites of reflection. The aorta and pulmonary trunk exit from the heart and are covered by pericardium for a distance of 2 or 3 cm. Ultrasound scans of the ascending aorta frequently show a linear density crossing the lumen that may simulate an obstruction of the aorta. A similar finding is present in normal neonates and infants who are being evaluated for coarctation of the aorta. The pericardial reflection from the left upper pulmonary veins creates a linear density that crosses the descending aorta below the level of the aortic isthmus.

DIAPHRAGM

The diaphragm can be evaluated from subcostal windows in transverse or sagittal scans. During scanning the movement of the right and left portions of the diaphragm can be visualized simultaneously (Fig. 12–2A). Normally the left portion is more inferior and is not as well silhouetted by the stomach as the right side by the liver. The diaphragm is traversed by the aorta, the inferior vena cava, and the esophagus. These entry sites or foramina are medial and are not mobile, so there is no differential movement at these sites. In sagittal, subcostal scans the descending aorta and its celiac and superior mesenteric branches can be seen. In such scans the left crus of the diaphragm is visualized routinely. It is a linear, relatively lucent structure in ultrasound scans and may be mistaken for a venous structure such as azygos continuation of the inferior vena cava (Figure 12–3).[4]

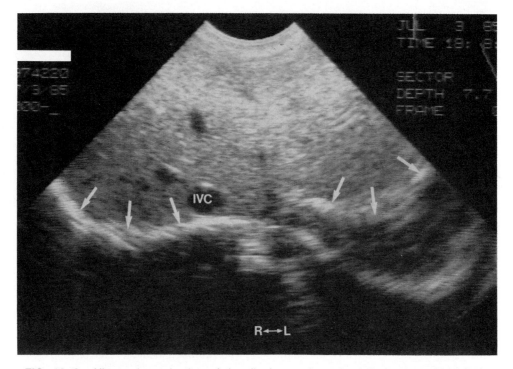

FIG. 12–2. Ultrasonic evaluation of the diaphragm from the subcostal approach in a transverse scan. The right and left diaphragms (white arrows) can be visualized moving normally from this approach.

ABNORMAL

PLEURAL EFFUSION

Fluid collections are the most common types of abnormalities of the pleura and pericardium. Large *pleural effusions* may completely surround the lung parenchyma, causing atelectasis. In this situation, ultrasound energy is transmitted throughout the thorax, and the collapsed lung segments can be imaged (Figure 12–4).

In addition to transudates of fluid into the pleural spaces, a large collection of blood *(hemothorax)* or chyle *(chylothorax)* will appear similar ultrasonically. Large pleural effusions of chylothorax may be diagnosed in the fetus by ultrasound imaging (Figure 12–5).

PERICARDIAL ABNORMALITIES

Large pleural effusions may make the diagnosis of pericardial effusion more difficult. The time-tested method used to distinguish pleural from pericardial fluid is to image the descending aorta.[5,6] In a long axis scan of the left ventricle,

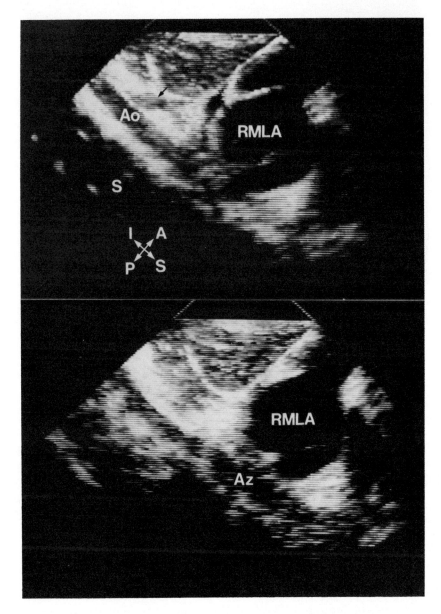

FIG. 12–3. Subcostal scans of a patient with azygos continuation (Az in lower panel) illustrating the crus of the diaphragm (black arrow in the upper panel). It is important not to confuse the crus with another venous structure.

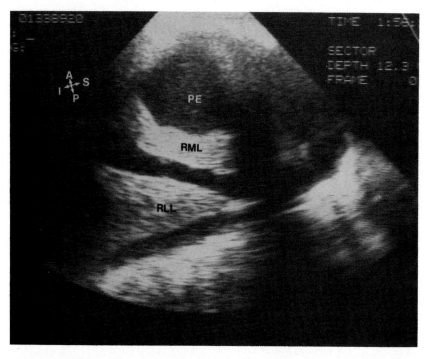

FIG. 12–4.   A sagittal scan of the right chest, which is filled with a pleural effusion (PE). The collapsed right middle lobe (RML) and right lower lobe (RLL) of the right lung are seen floating in pleural effusion.

the descending aorta is seen in cross-section. *Pericardial effusion* will extend anterior to the descending aorta but not behind the entire left atrium (Figure 12–6).

When pericardial effusion is large, an appearance on ultrasound scanning known as "the swinging heart" is produced. The heart is entirely encircled by a large amount of fluid. Observations of the pattern of movement of the right atrial and ventricular walls have shown a typical diastolic collapse when pericardial effusion compromises cardiac filling and produces tamponade.[7]

An area of atelectasis of the lung may accompany a fluid collection and simulate pericardial effusion (Figure 12–7).

Rarely, a defect in the pericardium or a *pericardial cyst* can cause an abnormal chest x-ray and be brought to medical attention.[8] In childhood, *partial absence of the pericardium*[9,10] may cause syncope or chest pain. Unusual rotation of the heart and abnormal cardiac position are features that should suggest the diagnosis.

Empty spaces around the heart may create confusion with blood-containing structures. Doppler ultrasonic techniques are useful to distinguish such empty spaces from abnormal vessels (Figure 12–8).

The finding of pericardial metastasis of extracardiac tumor is rare in childhood but has been detected by ultrasonography in the adult.[11]

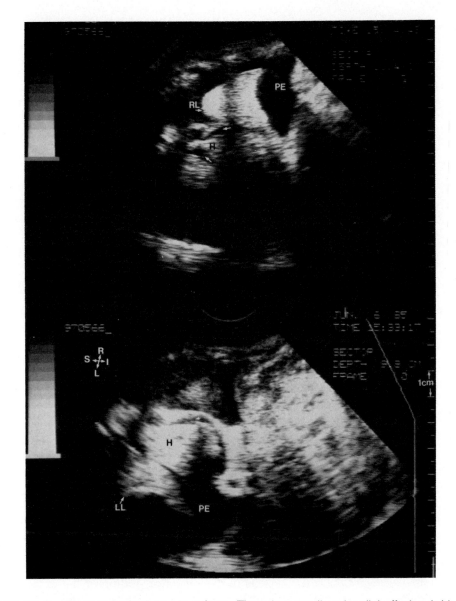

FIG. 12–5. Bilateral hydrothorax in a fetus. There is a small pericardial effusion (white arrows) and fluid surrounding both the right lung (RL) and the left lung (LL) (lower panel) H = heart.

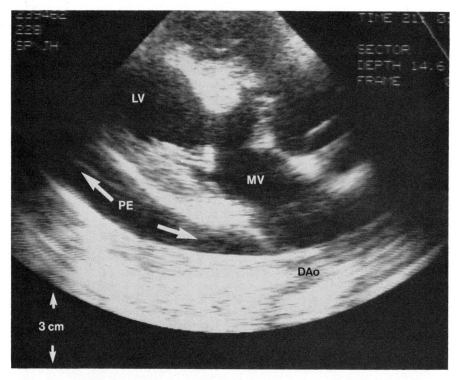

FIG. 12–6. A large pericardial effusion (PE) is recognized by an echolucency adjacent to the heart that passes anterior to the descending aorta (DAo). MV = mitral valve; LV = left ventricle; cm = centimeter.

DIAPHRAGMATIC ABNORMALITIES

The most common abnormality of the diaphragm is acquired paralysis caused by injury to the phrenic nerve. This can be evaluated readily by ultrasound imaging, which is quicker and more portable than fluoroscopy and does not entail ionizing radiation. The movement of the left and right portions of the diaphragm can be compared during inspiration and expiration (Figure 12–9). Left diaphragm paralysis may be more difficult to detect than right-sided dysfunction because the heart is resting on the left diaphragm, but inferior inspiratory motion usually can be imaged if adjacent stomach gas is not causing excessive ultrasonic reflections (Figure 12–10).

Congenital abnormalities of the diaphragm are rare but can be life-threatening, such as *diaphragmatic hernia*. Defects of the posterior portion of the diaphragm (Bochdalek's hernia) may result in herniation of the upper or lower gastrointestinal tract into the chest. There is a strong association with hypoplasia of the lung on the affected side and severe persistent pulmonary hypertension after birth. Ultrasonic scanning from the subcostal area can be used to image this type of defect.[12] An anterior defect (Morgagni's defect) may encroach on the inferior border of the heart (Figure 12–11). Such a defect may not be immediately recognized as a diaphragmatic hernia and may be falsely interpreted as a chest mass of another kind (see Chapter 13).

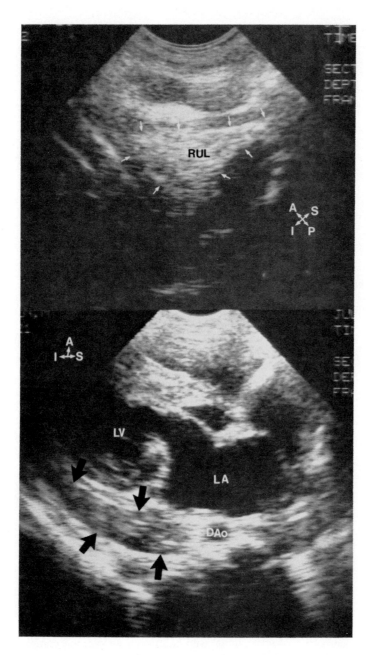

FIG. 12–7. Atelectasis of right upper lobe and left lower lobe in a patient with pulmonary disease. The collapse of the right upper lobe can be visualized with ultrasound imaging because of the lack of normal parenchymal aeration (upper panel). The left lower lobe (black arrows in the lower panel) was collapsed and simulated pericardial effusion because of its relative echolucency.

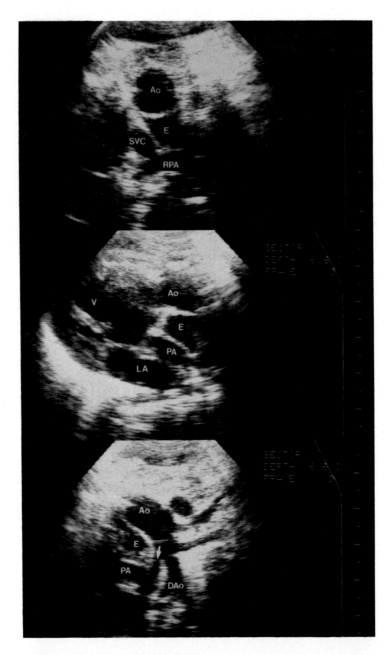

FIG. 12–8. Scans of a newborn infant with pulmonary atresia and complex congenital heart disease with an artifactual empty space (E) that caused initial confusion in the diagnosis. The aorta (Ao) and pulmonary artery (PA) are not adjacent but are separated by an echolucent area that is nonvascular, demonstrated by using Doppler ultrasound. On the suprasternal scan, the right pulmonary artery (RPA) was more inferior than normal (upper panel), making a palliative shunt more difficult to construct. The pulmonary arteries were confluent and supplied by a left patent ductus arteriosus (lower panel—white arrow). V = ventricle; SVC = right superior vena cava.

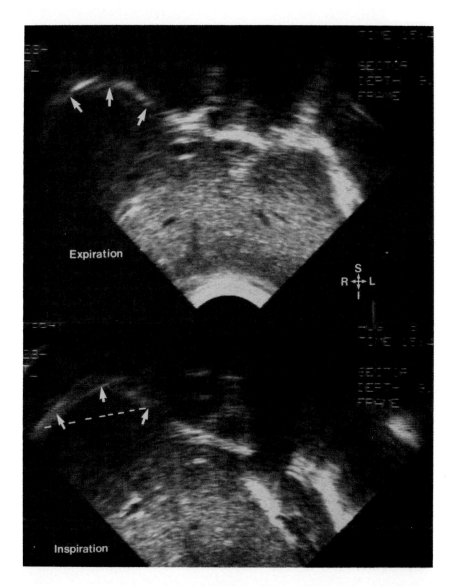

FIG. 12–9. Abnormal right hemidiaphragm that did not move inferiorly on inspiration. The dotted line shows the expected normal position of the diaphragm.

REFERENCES

1. Gutgesell HP, and Paquet M: Atlas of Pediatric Echocardiography. Hagerstown, MD, Harper & Row, 1978.
2. DCruz IA: Echocardiographic simulation of pericardial fluid accumulation by right pleural effusion. Chest 86:451, 1984.
3. DCruz IA: Echocardiographic simulation of pericardial effusion by ascites. Chest 85:93, 1984.
4. Huhta, JC, Smallhorn JF, and Macartney FJ: Cross-sectional echocardiographic diagnosis of azygos continuation of the inferior vena cava. Cathet Cardiovasc Diagn 10:221, 1984.
5. Popp RL, and Harrison DC: Echocardiography. In Noninvasive Cardiology, edited by AM Weissler. New York, Grune & Stratton, 1974, pp 149–226.
6. Silverman NH, and Snider AR: Two-Dimensional Echocardiography in Congenital Heart Disease. Norwalk, Conn, Appleton-Century-Crofts, 1982.
7. Armstrong WF, Schilt BF, Helper DJ, et al: Diastolic collapse of the right ventricle with cardiac tamponade: An echocardiographic study. Circulation 65:1491, 1982.
8. Hynes JK, Tajik AJ, Osborn MJ, et al: Two-dimensional echocardiographic diagnosis of pericardial cyst. Mayo Clin Proc 58:60, 1983.
9. Rowland TW, Twible EA, Norwood WI Jr, and Keane JF: Partial absence of the left pericardium. Diagnosis by two-dimensional echocardiography. Am J Dis Child 136:628, 1982.
10. Kansal S, Roitman D, and Sheffield LT: Two-dimensional echocardiography of congenital absence of pericardium. Am Heart J 109:912, 1985.
11. Friedman TD, Kotler MN, Victor MF, et al: Two-dimensional echocardiographic detection of pericardial and pleural metastases. J Cardiovasc Ultrasonography 1:205, 1982.
12. Kashani IA, Kimmons H, Valdes-Cruz LM, et al: Congenital right-sided diaphragmatic hernia and hypoplastic left heart syndrome. Am Heart J 109:177, 1985.

chapter **13**

EXTRACARDIAC
MASSES

Extracardiac masses in infants and children are rare but usually lead to thoracic exploration early in their evaluation because of the high incidence of treatable causes. Preoperative noninvasive evaluation of chest masses is performed by x-ray, computed axial tomography, and nuclear magnetic resonance imaging techniques. Little information is available regarding the use of ultrasound in the work-up of this problem in the pediatric age group. In adults, there are reports of echocardiographic recognition of most kinds of extracardiac tumors, including those of lymphatic, pericardial, vascular, enteric, and mesenchymal origins.[2-8] From these reports it is possible to characterize the areas where ultrasound imaging and Doppler interrogation may aid in the preoperative diagnosis of such masses when they are recognized at a young age. These areas include *localization* of the tumor with respect to adjacent cardiac structures, determination of whether the tumor is *solid versus cystic,* and identification of masses that are *vascular* or of cardiovascular origin.

In children the mediastinum and pericardium are rarely the site of metastasis because the tumors that commonly spread in this manner—including carcinoma of the lung, breast, and brain—are exceedingly rare in the younger age groups. In a recent review of 14 patients with *extracardiac masses* seen in the echocardiography laboratory at Texas Children's Hospital and confirmed pathologically over a three-year period, there were three with teratoma, four with aneurysm or pseudoaneurysm, two with lymphoma, and two with diaphragmatic hernia. Although they will not be discussed in detail here, during the same time period there were 26 patients with *intracardiac* tumors and more than 30 with other thrombi or masses inside the heart that could be visualized by ultrasound imaging.

LOCALIZATION

Extracardiac masses in children have been divided into two types based on their location in the anterior or posterior mediastinum. The anterior mediastinum extends from the suprasternal notch to the diaphragm and from immediately behind the sternum to a coronal plane through the hilus of the lung. The posterior mediastinum extends from the posterior, paravertebral gutters to the hilus (Plate XXIX).

ANTERIOR MEDIASTINAL TUMORS

The anterior mediastinum can be examined by parasternal, suprasternal, and subcostal scans. Masses immediately behind the sternum are in the near field of most commercially available ultrasound imaging systems, and adequate definition at shallow depths requires either high frequency transducers or special optimization for this purpose. At times it may be necessary to use a standoff over the chest, such as a bag containing ultrasound jelly, in order to place the region of interest in the focal distance of the transducer crystals.

The most common mass of the anterior mediastinum in a child is the *thymoma,* which is located in an anterosuperior position similar to the normal location of the thymus (see Chapter 4). Such a tumor may simulate cardiac tamponade and obstruction of the superior vena cava.[4] Another mass that may occur in a similar location and have a similar appearance is the cystic hygroma. Although cystic hygroma is usually confined to the neck, it may extend into the mediastinum and lie in the midline. Both of these entities may appear as echo-free masses, and differentiation from a dilated venous aneurysm may be possible with Doppler techniques (see further on).

A *teratoma* is a common mass of the chest in children that requires surgical treatment. It may present as a mass, but frequently it is adjacent to the heart and simulates cardiomegaly. Diagnosis is straightforward by finding an irregular mass with a distinct capsule separate from the pericardium (Figure 13–1). Pleural effusion may make the mass easier to identify (Figure 13–2).

A *diaphragmatic hernia* through the foramen of Morgagni creates an anterior space-occupying mass in the chest that may not be diagnosed readily in a critically ill infant or in a premature infant with other problems (see Figure 12–11).

Abscess formation may occur in the anterior mediastinum, particularly following a median sternotomy. Such a complication may begin as a postoperative hematoma[7] and progress to secondary infection (Figure 13–3).

POSTERIOR MEDIASTINAL TUMORS

Chest masses in the posterior mediastinum can be evaluated in children if an adequate pathway for ultrasound energy transmission is present because of the type, size, and location of the mass. For example, a large mass in the posterior mediastinum that makes contact with the diaphragm without intervening inflated lung tissue can be imaged from a subcostal approach because there is an "echo window" for this mass. If there is atelectasis of lung parenchyma, this will allow ultrasound imaging as long as there is no air obstructing the transmission of ultrasound energy. Good imaging also can be obtained in this situation when there is significant pleural fluid accumulation (Figure 13–4).

Lymphoma or *neuroblastoma* may occur in the most posterior portion of the posterior mediastinum and has a relatively homogeneous appearance (Figure 13–5). Such a mass may extend into the pericardiac area and may compress the left atrium or systemic veins.

The most common type of posterior diaphragmatic defect that creates herniation of abdominal contents into the posterior mediastinum is defect of the foramen of Bochdalek. If bowel contents herniate in the newborn, there may be severe respiratory distress requiring immediate surgery (Figure 13–6).

TISSUE CHARACTERIZATION—SOLID OR CYSTIC?

Tissue characterization by ultrasonography is in its infancy but has the greatest potential in children, in whom the imaging is superior and the ultrasound penetration is usually adequate. Masses can be categorized into those that appear

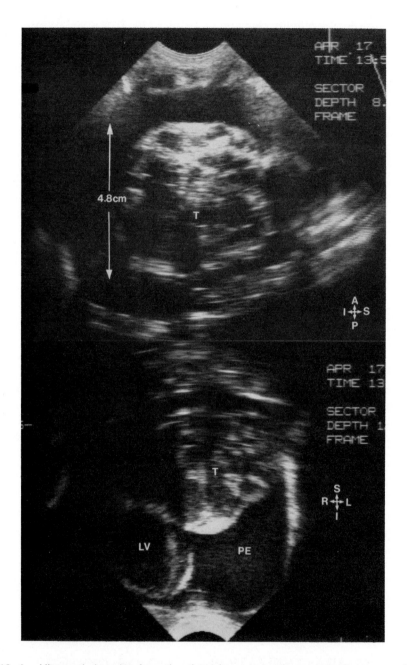

FIG. 13–1. Ultrasonic imaging from the chest (upper panel) and apex (lower panel) of a large teratoma (T). The mass was irregular and measured 4.8 cm in diameter. It was accompanied by a large pleural effusion (PE).

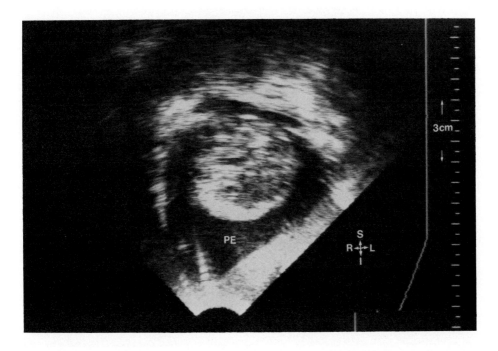

FIG. 13–2. Subcostal imaging of a large teratoma associated with pleural effusion. Note the enhanced echo imaging of the mass from the subcostal position as a result of the surrounding effusion.

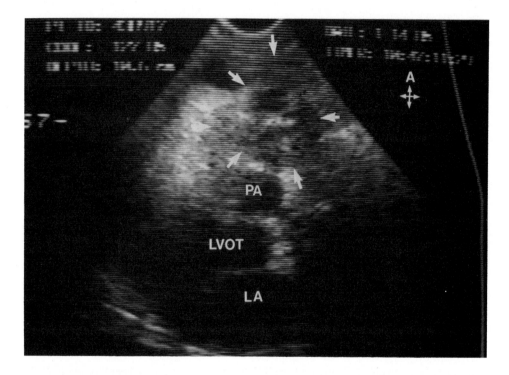

FIG. 13–3. Ultrasound imaging of the large anterior abscess (white arrows) in a patient with otherwise normal orientation of the pulmonary artery, left ventricular outflow tract and left atrium.

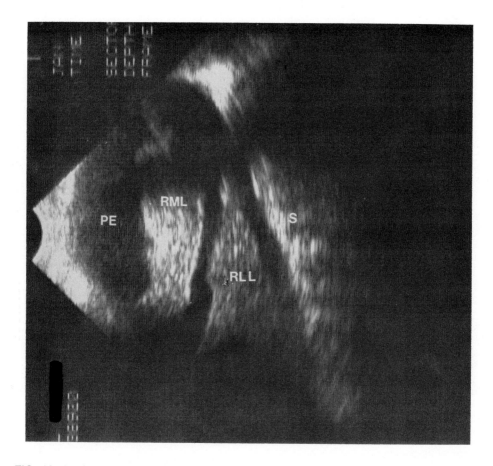

FIG. 13–4. Large pleural effusion with collapse of the right middle and right lower lobes of the lung. Sagittal scan shows the spine and the unusual imaging of the nonaerated lung attributable to the effusion.

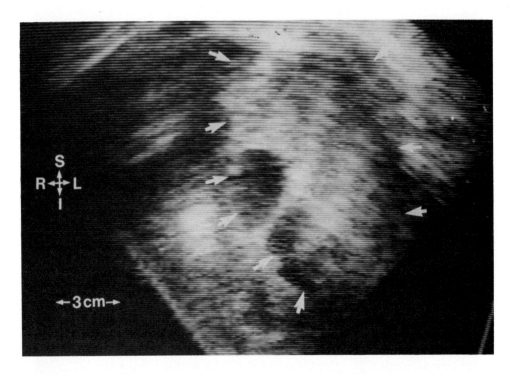

FIG. 13–5. Subcostal scanning of a large tumor mass (arrows) identified at surgery as a lymphoma. The mass was homogeneous, with the exception of two or three echolucent areas at its periphery.

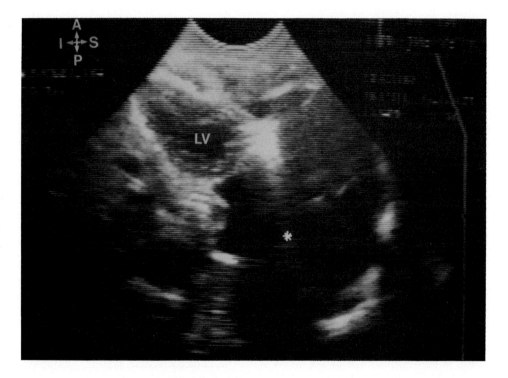

FIG. 13–6. Unusual finding in a patient with a diaphragmatic hernia and displacement of the bowel into the chest. The heart is well visualized and posterior to it is an air-containing mass (star).

(1) echolucent, (2) irregular with multiple cysts and echodensities, and (3) uniform with a monotonous granular ultrasound appearance. In the first category are the classic cystic masses discussed earlier, which include cystic hygroma, thymoma, and vascular aneurysms. The second type is exemplified by the teratoma, which has an appearance of multiple cysts and irregularities (see Figure 13–1). These tumors may contain hair and bone derived from embryonic tissues, giving them a very irregular appearance. There are many possibilities in the third type but, in children, the most common examples would be lymphoma and neuroblastoma.

Intracardiac tumors are dramatic, and ultrasound imaging is the diagnostic procedure of choice. At times the cardiac involvement of a tumor may be extensive, particularly in the case of *rhabdomyoma* in children (Figure 13–7). An example of an isolated tumor in the pulmonary artery is shown in Figure 13–8.

Masses in the vessels entering and leaving the heart are usually the result of indwelling catheters. A venous line used for intensive care monitoring may cause an extensive thrombosis of the inferior vena cava or leave an encasing sheath of fibrous tissue that remains even after catheter removal (Figure 13–9). In newborns, the umbilical arteries are used for arterial access, which may result in thrombosis in the descending aorta (see Chapter 7).

Infective endocarditis may occur outside the heart. A mass of infected tissue can occur at the site of turbulence created by a patent ductus arteriosus (Figure 13–10).

VASCULAR VS. NONVASCULAR—THE ROLE OF DOPPLER

The routine evaluation of a mediastinal mass in a child is inferential, utilizing noninvasive techniques for the most part, and it usually results in a differential diagnosis with a high likelihood of one lesion. Occasionally, however, the possibility of a vascular etiology of the mass gives pause to the thoracic surgeon, and cardiac catheterization is indicated. A technique that could confirm that there is communication of the mass with the cardiovascular system would be useful. Most often such a mass is the result of a complication of previous cardiovascular surgery, but there are examples such as *aneurysm of the ductus arteriosus* in which a relatively asymptomatic child could have a potentially life-threatening pulsatile mass.

Doppler ultrasonography has the potential to allow accurate diagnosis of such abnormalities (see Chapter 3). Detection of any blood flow velocity in the mass confirms the presence of the pulsatile flow in and out of the mass. If there is a history of enlargement of the mass on chest x-ray and if the clinical situation allows it, the patient should have cardiac catheterization and angiography prior to any surgery.

A vascular mass may simulate a pleural or pericardial effusion (see Chapter 12). Doppler sampling under imaging control can be used to confirm the presence of blood flow. Figure 13–11 shows a large left chest mass in a boy who had had previous cardiac surgery. There was a large *pseudoaneurysm* where blood had leaked from the region of the left ventricular outflow tract. In another case, an

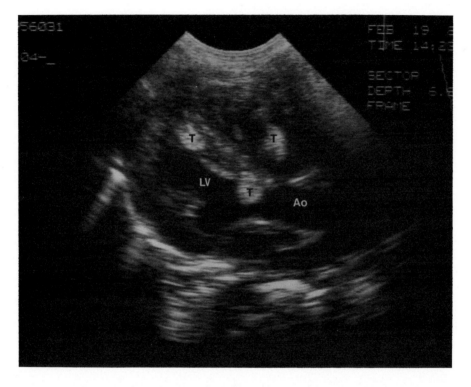

FIG. 13–7. Multiple tumor masses in a patient with tuberosclerosis and cardiac rhabdo-myomas. At least three tumor masses are seen on this parasternal scan of the left ventricle (LV) and aorta (Ao).

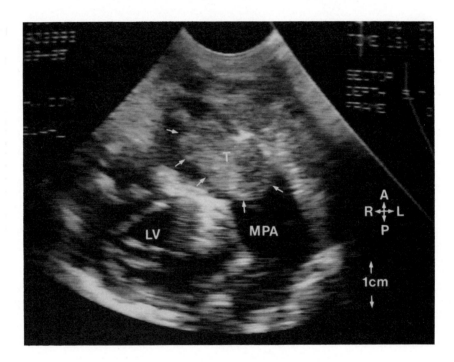

FIG. 13–8.   A large isolated sarcoma located in the main pulmonary artery (MPA). Such extracardiac masses may arise in an extracardiac structure, as was the case in this patient, or invade from other locations. (Reprinted with permission from the American College of Cardiology. J Am Coll 6:1362, 1985.)

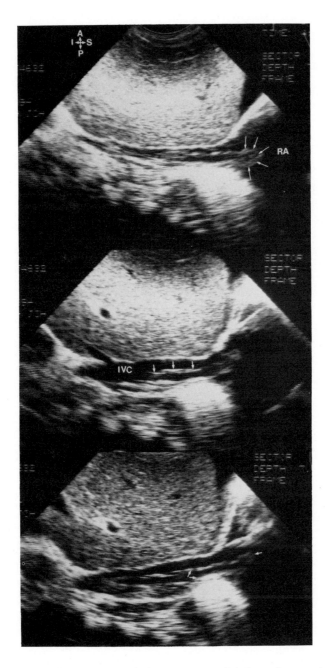

FIG. 13–9. Subcostal scans of the inferior vena cava showing a linear echolucency. Previous implantation and removal of a femoral venous catheter left a fibrous sheath with a mobile circular edge easily visualized in the right atrium (white arrows in the upper panel). The two parallel linear echodensities represent an encasement sheath of fibrous tissue that surrounded the catheter.

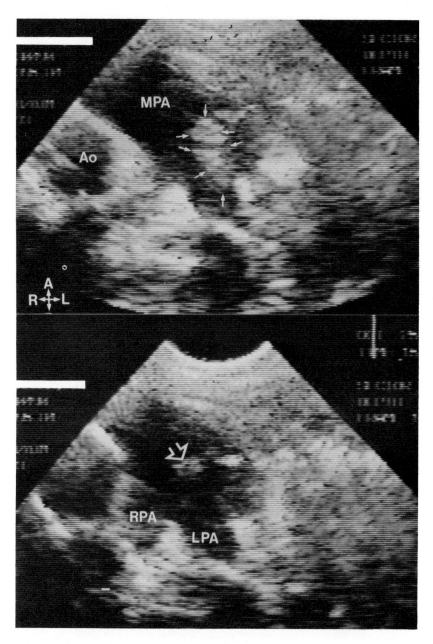

FIG. 13–10. High parasternal scanning of a vegetation in the main pulmonary artery caused by a patent ductus arteriosus in a 5-year-old child. There were clinical signs of subacute bacterial endocarditis, and this vegetation (white arrows, upper panel) was removed surgically. Postoperatively there was still residual vegetation in the main pulmonary artery (open white arrow in the lower panel).

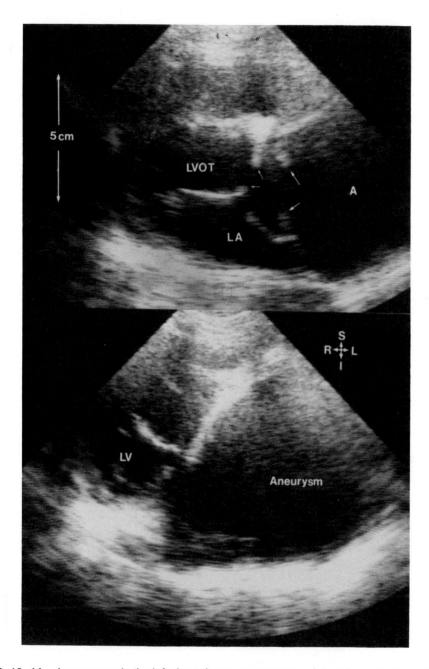

FIG. 13–11. Large mass in the left chest due to an aneurysm of the left ventricular outflow tract that freely communicated with the heart. The area of rupture of the heart into the aneurysm is shown by the white arrows in the upper panel.

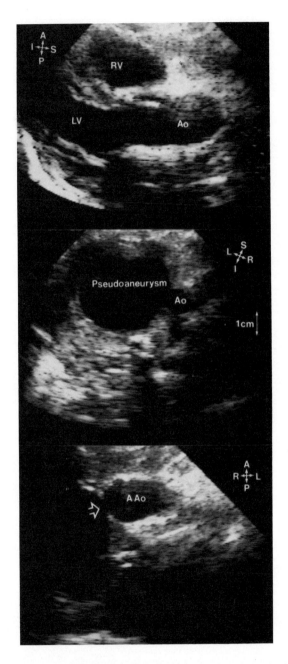

FIG. 13–12. Postoperative complication appearing in a patient who had repair of tetralogy of Fallot following an ascending aorta to right pulmonary artery shunt. The site of the previous Goretex® shunt created a pseudoaneurysm of the ascending aorta (middle panel). The site of opening of the pseudoaneurysm is shown in the lower panel.

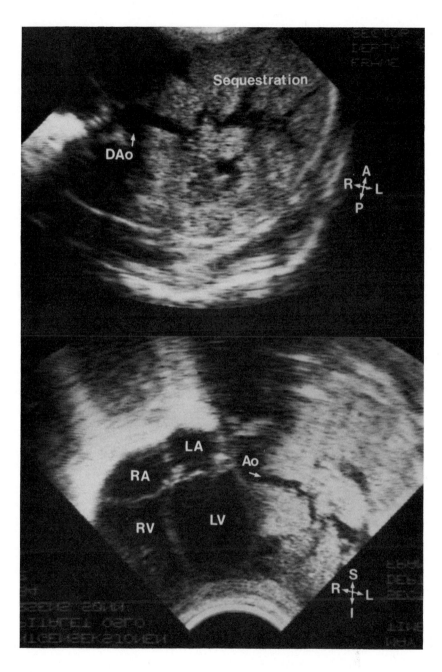

FIG. 13–13. Ultrasonic imaging of sequestration of the left lower lobe of the lung. The artery supplying the vascular mass from the descending aorta was well visualized (upper panel). An apical scan showed dilation of the left ventricle and again imaged the descending aortic feeder artery.

asymptomatic mass in the right side of the chest was caused by an ascending aortic aneurysm in a boy who had had previous palliative surgery (Figure 13–12).

A type of congenital vascular mass in the mediastinum is *sequestration*, which usually presents as a density on the chest x-ray. This is an abnormal segment of lung supplied by arteries from the descending aorta and frequently is associated with anomalies of pulmonary venous connection. The vascular aspect of such a mass in a newborn infant was confirmed by imaging the feeding arteries in one patient (Figure 13–13). The absence of normal left lower pulmonary venous connection was also defined (see Figure 10–6).

REFERENCES

1. Felner JM, and Knopf WD: Echocardiographic recognition of intracardiac and extracardiac masses. Echocardiography 2:3, 1985.
2. Chandraratna PAN, Littman BB, Serafini A, et al: Echocardiographic evaluation of extracardiac masses. Br Heart J 40:741, 1978.
3. Gottdiener JS, and Maron B: Posterior cardiac displacement by anterior mediastinal tumor. Chest 77:784, 1980.
4. Canedo MI, Otken L, and Stefadouros MA: Echocardiographic features of cardiac compression by a thymoma simulating cardiac tamponade and obstruction of the superior vena cava. Br Heart J 39:1038, 1977.
5. Tingelstad JB, McWilliams NB, and Thomas CE: Confirmation of a retrosternal mass by echocardiogram. J Clin Ultrasound 4:129, 1975.
6. Koch PC, Kronzon I, Winer HE, et al: Displacement of the heart by a giant mediastinal cyst. Am J Cardiol 40:445, 1977.
7. Gondi B, and Nanda NC: Two-dimensional echocardiographic diagnosis of mediastinal hematoma causing cardiac tamponade. Am J Cardiol 53:974, 1984.
8. Hynes JK, Tajik AJ, Osborn MJ, et al: Two-dimensional echocardiographic diagnosis of pericardial cyst. Mayo Clin Proc 58:60, 1983.

INDEX

Page numbers set in *italics* indicate figures; roman numerals indicate color plates.

221